THE 'Q' FACTOR

FACTOR

LIVING WITH AUTISM

Trudy Marwick

Trudy Marwick

Published by
Chipmunkapublishing
PO Box 6872
Brentwood
Essex CM13 1ZT
United Kingdom

http://www.chipmunkapublishing.com

Front cover design by Louise Sullivan.
http://www.louisesullivan.co.uk/

Chipmunkapublishing gratefully acknowledges the support of Arts Council England.

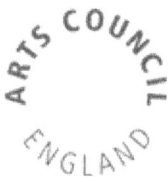

ARTS COUNCIL ENGLAND

THE 'Q' FACTOR

Chapters

Trudy Marwick

THE 'Q' FACTOR

Preface

Why the Q Factor?

What has the title got to do with Autism? Please read on and it might make sense…

The **Q factor** or **quality factor** compares the time constant for decay of an oscillating physical system's amplitude to its oscillation period. Equivalently, it compares the frequency at which a system oscillates to the rate at which it dissipates its energy.

This defination of the Q Factor is taken from Wikipedia, the free encyclopedia

Another use of the term is in bicycle terminology:

Q: What is this Q-factor thing?

A: Q-factor is a commonly used term which refers to the distance between the pedals.

This is taken from Sheldon Browns Bicycle Glossary.

I have chosen to use the term in the title for my book as I think it represents a little of what it is to be on the autistic spectrum. Ignoring the technical definitions of Q Factor and using it alongside popular current use of the term "X factor", then it makes sense. *X factor is a trademark of FremantleMedia Ltd. and Simco Ltd. Based on the television programme 'The X Factor' devised and owned by Simco and produced by talkback Thames.*

People on the Autistic Spectrum are different; we have an innate Q Factor. It is not about energy dissipation or anything to do with bicycles, but it is a factor or quality which is different. We do not have marketable appeal, star quality or typical iconic celebrity status as desired in the television programme The X Factor. We usually look totally ordinary, do not stand out in a crowd, except when we get things wrong socially and we do not usually desire fame. We may have some talents and exceptional abilities but these are not usually things the public crave.

The letter Q in scrabble is not usually a desirable letter. It scores 10 points which is the maximum for 1 letter on its own, but the Q always has to be laid in conjunction with a U and there are not as many word options available. Alone it cannot be used, and not with any other vowel but a U. However, the combination of a Q and a U along with other letters scores very highly. That is what I think it is like for people on the spectrum. People with ASD might have to be understood and accepted along with another person interpreting or explaining to them or for them. They may need someone to get alongside them, and break into their world – or unlock the autism. In isolation the person is not easily acceptable or able to fit in and help make a whole. Q is a unique and high scoring letter, but needing a U to unlock the potential. As in the game of scrabble, along with understanding and a link person, maximum points can be gained; the options might be more limited and it might be

THE 'Q' FACTOR

more difficult to fit into the whole, but the potential
for exceptional is there.
The Q Factor in my book refers to difference.

Introductions

Having a child with Autism brings challenges to life. It was while I was researching more about the subject so I could help my son that I first wondered if I was on the Autistic Spectrum myself. At first when I heard the word Autism I was frightened and unsure what the future would hold. I have been on a journey with my son through his development and I have learnt many lessons. He has changed my outlook and made me more accepting and tolerant of many people. He has shown me that his differences do not hold him back as he bravely faces challenges everyday. I have faced my own difficulties and am coming to terms with a diagnosis of Aspergers Syndrome. We have the Q Factor in our family, but rather than resent the difference, we embrace it as something special.

I am writing this book not as a professional with formal training on autism specifically, but as someone who has walked in the shoes for a few years now, and can share some things from a parent's perspective and personal experience.

Having lived with autism for a few years and researched the subject extensively makes me think I have something to write about. I would like to share some of our family's story in the hope that it might help other people who live with similar challenges. I started writing in preparation for a short talk on living with Autism Spectrum Disorder

THE 'Q' FACTOR

(ASD). Once I started writing, my thoughts were racing. I kept thinking of things I had to include to give a really good overview of what it is like living with someone on the spectrum. Then I began to add my own experiences as while I was preparing for the talk, I began my own journey towards diagnosis. The words flowed and the pages continued, it was no good as a talk anymore, but I carried on writing. When I had produced 10,000 words I thought I should abandon it as a talk but continue and see where it leads. I had to totally re write material for the talk or else my audience would have fallen asleep, but writing this book has been a truly cathartic experience.

Writing about my children has prompted memories of my own childhood. As I have sought to make sense of my son's world, it has helped me to understand my own. I hope my family will read this account and understand me better too, I do not think I have been an easy person to live with or to get to know. There have been misunderstandings and upsets, mistakes and trials. I think of my diagnosis as a way of understanding why I have always felt different. Throughout my life, especially in childhood, I did not feel accepted and I did not fit in.

Living with autism or with a child with autism is at times exciting, challenging, confusing, uncertain, scary, busy, lonely, rewarding but mostly exhausting.

I dedicate this book to my wonderful husband. Without his encouragement I would not have started this project nor had the strength to complete it.

I am also grateful to my parents who have been enduringly patient and have loved me despite the odds, accepted my "prickly" ways and been there through the hard times.

To my children I have to say a huge thank you as they have taught me so much over the years, given me the material to write, the laughter and the tears. Their stories will continue and I do not know the ending, but I know there are adventures along the way.

THE 'Q' FACTOR

What is autism?

Text books state that:
Autism is a lifelong developmental disability that affects the way a person communicates and relates to people around them. Children and adults with autism have difficulties with everyday social interaction. Their ability to develop friendships is generally limited as is their capacity to understand other people's emotional expression.

"Reality to an autistic person is a confusing, interacting mass of events, people, places, sounds and sights. There seems to be no clear boundaries, order or meaning to anything. A large part of life is spent just trying to work out the pattern behind everything."

What are the characteristics of autism?
People with autism generally experience three main areas of difficulty; these are known as the triad of impairments.

- **Social interaction** (difficulty with social relationships, for example appearing aloof and indifferent to other people)
- **Social communication** (difficulty with verbal and non-verbal communication, for example not fully understanding the meaning of common gestures, facial expressions or tone of voice)
- **Imagination** (difficulty in the development of interpersonal play and imagination, for example having a limited range of

imaginative activities, possibly copied and pursued rigidly and repetitively).
The text book definition is easy to find on the internet or in the many helpful books written by the experts, but I would like to write about some stories about home life and how we cope day to day living with autism.

Diagnosis

I couldn't write a book like this without mentioning Diagnosis. Finding the reason why a child is different is important. Having a label gives a benchmark for understanding. You can start to read and learn about the condition and how it affects your child. Some people might cling to a label and possibly limit the abilities of their child. I have learnt that my children all do things which are way beyond my expectations. They constantly surprise me with their abilities and also their difficulties.

Months can go by when we forget we are living with "labels" but we just see the children and accept them as they are. Then something crops up to remind us of the difficulties and challenges our children face and we revisit the diagnosis which helps make sense of things and hopefully find a positive way through the difficulty.

In order to get that all important diagnosis, you have to invite many professionals into your family. Living with someone who is different means that your private world is open to scrutiny. Every detail is examined and considered. You tell the same stories over and over again. In the search for diagnosis, every fact is considered and as a parent you can't help feel guilt that you have a child who is different. Should I have eaten differently when pregnant, was it the drugs they used while in labour, should I have put the baby to sleep in a different position? These are just some of the random questions that go through your mind and guilt is passed about. Is there a genetic reason? Does it come from my family or his? Will other children be affected? It goes on and on.

Life with a child with any disability is full of psychological assessments, tears, medical investigations, tears, benefit forms, tears, meetings with professionals, tears, reviews, tears, targets, therapists, procedures, invasive procedures, care plans etc etc. So as a parent you have to be comforter, teacher, advocate, business manager, clinician, interpreter, medical expert, nurse, physio, OT, dietician, life coach, mentor, scribe, personal assistant, gopher, and friend to name but a few!

But the most important thing is not to forget the CHILD! It can become too easy for people to forget the person and just look at the label.

Things at the beginning.
I knew my son was different at the age of 2 when he still didn't speak and he had only just learnt to walk, by the age of 2 ½ we used to go to the local play group and Ben was the only one not playing with other children. When it was time for an activity and all the children would be lining up for snack or to go outside, Ben would be driving a train on the table around the edge of the room or spinning the wheels and watching them.

THE 'Q' FACTOR

At 3 ½ I can remember having to leave toddler groups early when my son would start a trend in behaviour. The children would be happily playing, then someone would notice Ben playing under the stacks of spare chairs and thinking it looked fun. A trail of other 3 year olds and little baby brothers and sisters would climb under the chairs too. You can imagine, not a safe place for the entire gang of kids to hang out and certainly from Ben's point of view – too many people! He would let rip with his now familiar high pitched shriek and start chaos! It would be worse if a child tried to share the toy Ben was playing with, he would pull it away from the other child until it ended in tears.

Crying children ran to mums, mums gave me the hard stare, I would grab Ben, coats and bag, make a few hasty apologies and leave! I think I tried a few different groups, but when you arrive and the room goes quiet, or you hear the remainder of a comment like – that's **that boy!** It becomes clear that although the sign says, everyone welcome, you realise, autism is not!

So at 3 ½ feeling my sons development was definitely not following a "normal" pattern, we went to a health visitor who did a hearing test and then referred us to another health visitor, who referred us to a GP who referred us to a speech therapist who referred us to a paediatrician who gave us a social worker. I began to get used to watching my son fail the assessments, not understand what was expected of him and watch him get very upset by it all. Months of long meetings, giving the same information each time, assessments and stress followed and then I heard the words.

"Your son has autism. There is no cure; he won't grow out of it. He might be able to go to a special school where they might be able to teach him to speak, but he won't fit in".

So, I read as much as I could about autism and watched Rainman again and braced myself to tell family and friends – the few I had left. Even close family have taken a few years to cope with the diagnosis and they have changed their opinions gradually. At first one sister said, do you think it was your divorce which caused it? He'll grow out of it wont he?

One friend asked, "will you put him in a home? How will you cope"?

There was much denial, embarrassment, and few invitations. We might cause a scene? Show the family up? Have a tantrum at the wrong moment?

I am glad to say, that we have survived it all and now, I wouldn't change my son for a moment. I have to admit to you that I haven't always felt like that. In the early days after diagnosis I sometimes wished there was a switch which could be flicked in his brain which would change it all. I went through a kind of bereavement process for the son

THE 'Q' FACTOR

I thought I had and gradually began to get to know the son who I am blessed with.

I even wished his disability was more physical so he could be included and accepted a bit more. I am glad to say that in 15 years a lot has changed and now people with autism are much more understood.

So all that was before the official label, and before there was so much publicity about autism, have things changed? The circumstances have changed, but the problem is still there. We still have the child who is different and who can show that "inappropriate or challenging behaviour" you never know when it is about to happen!

Diagnosis for me was also not a straightforward process. In an attempt to understand my son better, I read all I could on autism and watched countless documentaries and films about it. It was while reading Luke Jackson's book "Freaks, Geeks and Aspergers Syndrome" that I started to feel that I was really reading about my own childhood. I could identify with most of what he wrote, the misunderstandings, difficulties decoding social situations and expectations, constantly feeling different and odd. All my life I have been desperately trying to find answers. Why do I constantly feel out of place socially, and why I have such difficulty making friends and maintaining relationships. I read more books, researched what I could on the internet about adult diagnosis of AS (Aspergers Syndrome), and I realised I was not the only person who as an adult had Aspergers which was not diagnosed in childhood.

After digging about on the internet and pointers from the National Autistic society I found an online test for Aspergers Syndrome. It is the AQ test designed by Simon Baron Cohen and colleagues at Cambridge Autism Research Centre. I did the test many many times, and I still do the test regularly to see if I have grown out of my difficulties! I scored 47 and it suggests that Eighty percent of those diagnosed with autism or a related disorder scored 32 or higher. The test is not a means for making a diagnosis, however, and many who score above 32 and even meet the diagnostic criteria for mild autism or Aspergers report no difficulty functioning in their everyday lives.

So I did the test, read the books, understood myself more than I have ever done and could rationalise many painful memories. To me, the fact I understand I am different has helped me accept myself more. I started to think more positively about myself. I still have moments of self doubt and feel pain and anxiety on a daily basis when I know I get things wrong socially. But I could get on with things knowing there is a reason why I have some difficulties.

THE 'Q' FACTOR

After 3 years trying to come to terms with the fact that I think I have AS, a local professional came to work with my daughter and help us support her with some difficulties she was having at school. I sat with my daughter watching her being tested for dyslexia type difficulties. I struggled with many of the tests myself and my answers were totally different to my daughter's who came out with abilities functioning way above her age group, but the tests showed some areas where her development is behind. This gave us an understanding of why she was having difficulty with some school work and the school also took the results of the assessments and used them to find ways to support my daughter's learning. This was a very happy outcome for Lauren, she could see that she has some difficulties, but she is also doing very well and understanding at an age much older than her years. She was compensating for her difficulties very well but now she can be given more help.

During the assessments, I had the opportunity to discuss some of the difficulties I have and it was the understanding and acceptance of what I was saying about possibly having AS which gave me the confidence to try and formally get a diagnosis. I am very grateful to the lady who helped me feel the confidence to formalise a diagnosis. And I am also thankful to a local well respected professional. He came to a training event about autism, to speak to a group of parents about his work and the service he provides and he said to us that he has AS himself - that also helped make me feel confident enough to try and "go public."

I took my story and the AQ test results to the local Principal Educational Psychologist. I asked for a meeting with her to discuss some issues about my son, and also asked if I could talk to her about the feeling that I might have AS myself.

She listened to my story and reviewed the test. She assured me that Simon Baron Cohen is extremely well regarded in the field of autism research and that the AQ test would therefore be a reliable tool for use around diagnosis of Autistic Spectrum Disorder. She said that I could leave the meeting with her, with the understanding that she agreed with my thoughts that I have AS. With this knowledge I could just get on with life as before, I would not be any different, other than I could better understand some areas of difficultly. However, she also told me the route to take to establish a formal diagnosis as in her role; she is not qualified to formally diagnose adults.

To me this was another step in the right direction (to use a figure of speech I do understand!) She had not rubbished my opinion and belief about myself, and showed me respect and value. She asked if I would be prepared to speak about my experience as it might help teachers and professionals understand and support children hearing the story from an adult. The thought of speaking in public is not something I feel comfortable about, but I was grateful for her showing confidence in me.

My long suffering husband and I had talked for hours about whether or not I could have AS. He said that he felt it made sense of a lot of times when I would misunderstand him totally and often feel hurt without due cause. It made sense of how I struggled with work situations when faced with new and daunting projects or tasks. He was the person who was with me and supporting me through tears and self doubt. He helped me when I felt I had been bullied at work, gave me advice on how to handle people. He managed to do all of this without making me feel inadequate for which I am very grateful.

I read "born on a blue day" by Daniel Tammet. Again I felt I could identify with some of his memories about his childhood. I also read "Thinking in Pictures" by Temple Grandin. Both books are totally honest accounts of their lives and their exceptional talents and abilities. I got a great amount of comfort from the books because it helped me accept myself. Both authors are exceptional people who make a wonderful contribution through their insights and knowledge. Obviously I do not feel that I am blessed with their wonderful talents but I do know I have some abilities which are different to people around me. Reading the books helped me accept my differences and feel more positive about them. Both authors do not feel sad that they are different, but celebrate the fact that they can be themselves in a world which gives them challenges every day, the books also celebrate their uniqueness.

The next step for me was to discuss things with my GP and request a consultation with a clinical psychologist. I had the opportunity to explain to the Doctor why I felt it was necessary for me to get a formal diagnosis. It does not change the way I am or give me a cure or make me better or worse. It is not a negative step, but I feel a formal diagnosis gives me the confidence and the credibility to speak about something I understand and experience. It also gives me the confidence to ask when I do not understand something, and the knowledge that I am asking the question not because I am stupid but because I have some difficulties processing language and social situations. I can ask for implied meanings and ask what is expected of me, not because I am lazy and cannot be bothered to think for myself, but because these are some of the things I do not automatically understand.

I am not keen to get a label for the sake of it, for me it means I can say with some authority that I have some differences, I have some strengths but also some areas of difficulty. I feel now that if I am in a situation where I am not able to access the information, I will say that. If the format or information is not easy for me to understand, I will ask the necessary questions with the knowledge

THE 'Q' FACTOR

that I am not "stupid" but I have difficulty decoding some phrases.

To explain what I mean; in meetings I find it very tiring and frustrating when you have to decode unnecessary jargon and abbreviations. I lose the place in the talk or conversation as I am systematically decoding the phrases word by word and then visiting the filing cabinet of phrases I have in my head and pulling out the time a kind person explained the phrase as a whole to me and reading it in my head. I can see the words as a picture of a book in my head, a kind of dictionary. I can turn the pages and see the lists of jargon I have learnt or figures of speech I have had explained to me. While I am doing this, the talk has obviously moved on and I have lost the place. I have started to admit in meetings now that I have "lost the plot" at what ever place I found I had reached mental overload through trying to decode and process the information which was not in an accessible format for me. I used to smile with others and laugh on cue following other people in the group or conversation. I would then later spend time trying to decode the part of the conversation I could not understand and make sense of the whole again. This is a tiring process and often leaves me behind in social contexts.

As with figures of speech, with abbreviations I have to mentally decode the abbreviations letter by letter and fill the gaps next to the letter with the word it represents. This is again done in pictures,

I have a picture of another book in my head, a sort of encyclopaedia with lists of letters and abbreviations and the definitions next to them. While I am reading and sorting pages the letters I can see in my head I sometimes get distracted from the flow of the talk or conversation. While I am trying to understand the abbreviations in the context of the current conversation, my brain can't help reading the same letters and trying to remember the abbreviation in another context and relate internally why it is totally inappropriate to rely on these abbreviations as they are so misleading. To use a simple example AA in one context means alcoholics anonymous and automobile association in another!

Despite telling lecturers and fellow students on my university course that I find it very difficult to decode abbreviations and figures of speech, they were used all the time. I would constantly lose my place in the conversation or during a lecture because I would be stuck on decoding the letters of the abbreviation or trying to understand what "steel fist in a velvet glove" or "pig in a poke" mean and why it was at all relevant to use that in the current situation!

After most meetings and times of concentration such as lectures, sermons, talks, conversations or watching TV, I actually get a head ache and have to go somewhere quiet and unravel the tread of thoughts in my head.

THE 'Q' FACTOR

I have found it is particularly useful to have handouts at the beginning of a seminar or meeting. This is actually difficult as speakers are often worried about handing out literature or printouts of slides as they worry people will be so busy reading ahead or looking up answers that it is not helpful. I find I have to ask specifically for the handouts and explain that it is useful for me to have them as I can annotate them and it helps me to see the information in front of me. I can look back at pages and refresh my memory about the abbreviations relevant to that talk or the technical terms used. I was advised to say I am a bit dyslexic as that seems an appropriate way of explaining why I need the handouts, I would prefer it however if it was understood as being useful to more people and that we are not going to use them as a way to cheat or day dream away the seminar. It just really helps me see where the talk is going in a visual way and I scribble over the handouts so it helps me remember. It is difficult as you have to put your hand up and admit that you are a bit different and that you need the information in a different way to other people, but when I am able to have the handouts at the beginning to follow through the seminar or meeting, it makes a huge difference to me. I went to a National Autistic Society (NAS) seminar recently and they handed out the papers at the beginning, it felt as if I had won the lottery, I was so thrilled that I got the information I needed without having to ask for it and admit I am different in front of a room full of people I hardly know. I hope this will be a trend taken up by many organisations as more is learnt about Autistic Spectrum Disorder.

So to me obtaining a diagnosis of AS was very important, it gives me the confidence to ask the questions I need to ask to be able to understand and access the world around me. I ask many questions of my husband when I do not understand something, I am so thankful to him because he has helped me keep up with the plot of my favourite TV programmes or films, he also explains figures of speech to me, the meanings of jokes and also the implied meanings I miss most of the time. He now understands why I have to ask the questions, he does not belittle me or tease me or imply that I am stupid. I trust him so I can open up to him and show my areas of difficulty. I was not always so fortunate, as admitting that you do not understand or that you need help understanding some things which are so obvious to others can be a sure way of being ridiculed and belittled. Sadly there are some people who take great delight in proving they have superior intellect to others. I do not now see my difficulties as part of an inferior intellect, but as a difference in how I process information.

I do not think that diagnosis is important just for the sake of having a label, it does not make a person any different, but it helps understand them. I believe a label of AS gives me an association with others who have ASD. I believe that if I have

THE 'Q' FACTOR

some difficulties, then others with ASD may possibly experience the same or similar difficulties. I think it is therefore important for someone like me, to tell their story and to do so in the hope that it might make things easier for others who for what ever reason cannot or do not wish to tell their story.

Childhood memories

In my journey to finding a diagnosis, I had to revisit many childhood memories. The books I read reminded me of painful experiences in my childhood. 1 of 5 children, I felt I had a lonely childhood. I was happier on my own pursuing my own interests or playing along side my siblings, but not really playing with them. I was very good at directing games; my younger sisters would patiently play lego with me. My interest was to make the lego people, line them up and name them in family groups. Usually mum, dad and 3 children. I preferred to have 3 girls in my typical family group. I would then make a house, organise the furniture until I was happy with it and then line up my family in the house, or in front of it as if they were visitors. I would sit alongside my sisters changing the furniture and fiddling with the people to straighten their arms or align their hair. By this time, my sisters would be in an imaginary game playing with the people, quite happily in the house I had made them, or they would copy the formula of the game on their own. Make the people, name them, make a house and play the game. I could only seem to get as far as make the house and got stuck on the play the game part.

This is one of my happy childhood memories. I believed I was playing with my sisters, but looking back, I was directing my sisters who were happy to comply. I would get frustrated when they played the game and it disturbed the order in my house or in the part of the house I was using. Then I used to get stressed and possibly destroy their fun by breaking my family and putting the lego away. I would go off to do something else and my 2 sisters would often carry on playing together quite happily. I did not really need to be part of the game for them at all. I used to think this was because I am 2 years older than my nearest sister and she is closer in age to our younger sister than in age to me. Therefore it is logical that they should get on well together. I can now see that the real logic is that they find relating to other people easier than I do and they are more comfortable in the company of others, they are more sociable and easier to get along with. They are able to play with someone else, rather than play alongside someone, without actually sharing their game which is what I seem to do.

My 2 sisters nearest in age to me both had a special friend when they were young, I envied this very much. My youngest sister is 10 years younger than me and so when I moved away from home at the age of 17, she was only 7. For much of her child hood, I was not living there. So I do not remember her childhood patterns of play and friendships in the same way.

I did not have a special friend for any length of time. My sisters seemed to be able to maintain friendships. They had invitations to sleep over at a friend's and also had friends to stay. I did not.

In primary school I do not remember friendships lasting longer than a few months, and certainly not beyond academic years into the next class. I remember the playground as a difficult place. I preferred to stay in and do jobs for the teacher. I also got very good at taking my time so that I did not finish a task before break. Then I would be allowed to stay in at play time until I had completed the activity. I used to finish my work and then sit on the pipes in the cloakroom unnoticed until the bell rang after play. I could then join the line of children and wait to go into class. I spent many happy hours sitting alone on the pipes following the patterns of pipes and wires on the ceiling in the cloakroom. I counted the coat pegs, counted the number of gym shoes in the pockets under the pegs and worked out who had forgotten to bring their lunch box in that day by the gaps in lunch boxes on the pegs. In those days, we used to have the option of going home for dinner. I preferred to do that each day and as my Mum was usually home we could take that option, it meant we could time our lunch time so that we didn't have a long period of time at play in the playground but arrive just in time for the bell to go.

If I was out in the playground, I found it difficult. Some days we used to play big games like "what's the time Mr Wolf?" That was easier as there were rules and a structure, I just joined in if I was allowed. I used to hang about at the edge of the playground and look for stag beetles. I mention them later in the section on collecting.

THE 'Q' FACTOR

I found making friends with some of the boys easier than the girls. I am a fairly good mimic (in common with many people with ASD), so I could relate to 2 boys in the class who were keen comedy performers. They based their performances on the Mike Yarwood show and did characters accordingly. I was allowed to join them as my impression of Margaret Thatcher was more passable than any of the other girls. It gave me a few pleasant play times as we rehearsed for performance. I don't think we were likely to be picked for "New Faces" but it was a short friendship activity which I enjoyed.

Music

My mother recently reminded me that I taught other children to play the recorder just so that I had others to play music with. Once I had a grasp of an instrument, it was like a ticket into social activity. Our teacher taught recorder and I took it very seriously. I soon got better than other children my age who were more interested in making "train whistle noises" as my teacher described them. I was given a tenor recorder and because I have large hands I was able to play fairly easily. I love the sound it makes and practised for hours at a time. I tried to find others who wanted to play duets or in groups, but this did not happen until secondary school.

I like being part of a group of musicians. I like to contribute to a whole sound. I am not a soloist by choice, but will at times play exposed parts in a whole piece. But always with another instrument playing, so I am not alone.

In music groups, there is an etiquette which I feel comfortable with. You have a ticket into the group as you carry an instrument. You fit in, and do not have to explain yourself, you can sit down next to people who you don't know but you don't have to talk to them other than pass comments about the conducting or conversation about the music. It is a structured environment which is comfortable for me.   You know what is expected of you and it is easy to join in. It is usually directed by a

THE 'Q' FACTOR

conductor or a music leader which gives a comfortable structure to practice sessions. Being part of a group, there is a pressure as you have to practice the music or else it is obvious that you are the one who cannot play at the right time. I find that difficult as I do not cope well with pressure, but I enjoy the music so much that I have always tried to play along with other people. I am not very creative, so I usually prefer to read the music and play as written, I find it more challenging if expected to improvise, but that is also something you can learn to do. There are rules to follow, so it becomes easier, I also copy what I hear others play and use that as a basis for my own contributions.

I do find performance challenging as I get very nervous. I prefer the practise sessions to the performance. Sometimes I get so nervous my mouth goes dry and my arms and legs shake. I am better if I try to relax and think that the performance is no big deal. I am a perfectionist so set high standards for myself. I will not be happy unless I have played note perfect. I do not do that very often, but usually the last practice before the event is my best moment and I am happy with that. The pressure of the performance and the nerves take over during the concert and I make mistakes and miss entries in the music I know I can usually play very easily. Because of nerves sadly I am not as aware of the musicality. I am not so able to listen to others around me and focus on playing the music as a whole; I am so focused on managing to get through without making the mistakes and concentrating on my own playing. I watch the conductor and follow them, but am not so aware of the sound as a whole. I am not the best musician but I do enjoy being part of music making. After a recent concert, I was told I was staring intently at the conductor and they found it unnerving. I find it easy to memorise large sections of the music and so often I will watch the beat of the conductor. I can see the music as a picture in my head, so for me it is easy to follow the beat and the music at the same time. I do find the rules of eye contact difficult, I try to take any comments from others and learn from them, so I will try to ensure that I am watching the conductor, but hopefully not making them nervous in the process. Making eye contact is something I have to consciously think to do, but I have also learnt it is equally important to break the eye contact intermittently. This is something which is not automatic or natural; I have to consciously move my gaze and look at something else and then return my eye contact to the person. In the orchestra or music group, I watch the conductor if I need to follow their beat for a part of the music or if someone else in the orchestra has difficulty playing in time and I need to follow the beat more than listen to the other player. I have now learnt that I need to break the eye contact so that the conductor is not offended by my intent stare.

THE 'Q' FACTOR

I recently tried my first session at a local music venue. It was fun but I found it daunting that no one uses music. They all know the tunes (traditional music) and can play really well, my musical ear is not really good enough to contribute much to such a sound, but it was enjoyable having a go at a true "jam session" with true folk musicians. Music is a way for people to join in socially even thought they might find social situations very difficult.

My children are all musical. Nick chooses football and sport over music, but Ben and Lauren are both learning instruments. Ben has perfect pitch. He can play by ear and will hear a tune and can play it back on the fiddle or pick it out with on the keyboard. I have some pitch abilities to a degree, I can hear the correct note in my head when I am familiar with a piece of music, but Ben can hear the note and tell you what it is and what key the piece of music is in. He does not know the names of the keys, but tells you how many black notes it has and which note it starts on. That is sufficient evidence to know that he can hear the pitch of the notes but the technical ability to relate those notes to the conventional name of the key is something he can be taught.

At school I went to everything possible to do with music, I joined the choir both junior and senior (at the same time). I was in recorder ensembles, groups and chamber groups, orchestra, and helped younger pupils in practice "sessions" or took the junior orchestra when I out grew it. If music activities were cancelled, I was totally at a loss during my lunch time. I found the time before school and break time very difficult. I used to walk to my next lesson and hang about outside the classroom, or just walk around the school until the next lesson was about to start. As I don't like to be late, I was careful to time my walking about so that I was always in the right place before the bell rang.

I can remember utter confusion when the school introduced a one way system. It challenged my use of time at break, as now I had to walk in one direction and this meant I did not have time to wander in the same way as you had to go around an entire block before you got back to the classroom. I think schools cope much better with people with AS now, as sometimes rooms are set aside for people who need quiet and structure to go and wait until the next lesson. One of our local schools has a wonderful librarian who makes the library open to people who need a quiet place during breaks. She is so aware of the difficulties some pupils have with social times that she also gives tasks such as cataloguing books or helping put books back on the shelves. She runs the chess club and provides an invaluable service to many pupils on the autistic spectrum and others who are not on the spectrum but for other reasons like a quiet structured environment.

THE 'Q' FACTOR

Music is a way for me to join in socially, it provides me with a structured environment. I also find it is a way to express emotions. Sometimes I cannot name the emotion I am feeling, but if I feel sad or frustrated, I will often play some music. I am not very good at describing how listening to music makes me feel or music appreciation. My daughter Lauren is very good at describing what the music makes her imagine. I can remember music lessons where we were expected to listen to a piece of music and describe what it was about. I found it easy to see a picture in my head of what I thought the music was about, but it was usually totally different to anyone else's descriptions or what the composer actually intended. I enjoy watching ballet as it is a visual way of understanding the music. The dancers interpret the music and bring it to life.

The trouble with undiagnosed Aspergers syndrome

I am glad to have found out why I am different. I have been so aware all my life that I do not fit in easily. I have heard the expression "school days are the best days of your life" but I do not believe that at all. Sadly school days for people who are not diagnosed in childhood are more likely to be traumatic and full of sad memories. Teenagers with undiagnosed AS are more likely to experience depression and other mental health difficulties.

Having watched day time TV with shows such as Oprah or Trisha, I have often wondered by people feel the need to "go public" on national TV and expose their most intimate secrets. Writing this feels a little like that. I am revealing weaknesses and sharing difficulties, but I am now confident that the difficulties I have had are not due to weakness of character. I have not always felt that.

As a teenager, I always felt very different. I did not get invited out with friends very often. I can remember going to the cinema with a group of girls on one occasion, but that was only thanks to one girl in a group of friends who kindly included me in her invitations. I did get invited to friends houses, but usually only once. I did invite friends to my house, but again this did not happen often. Friendships did not last long. I remember one friend coming to our home to revise for an exam,

THE 'Q' FACTOR

she came once but I never got invited to her home. I remember revising and reading the text book while she was there, but I don't think she wanted to study, I could not think what else we were going to do? Just "hanging out" with friends did not seem easy to me.

It is possible that I did not have the same interests as other girls my age. I was interested in the music of James Galway, and listened to his records and not pop music until much later than my classmates. I did not know how to relate to boys. My relationship with my brother meant I was used to being teased. I was close to my brother in my late teens, but until then I was wary of boys as I had been bullied or teased by them. I was always the kid who had the snow balls hurled at them or their bag thrown off the bus.

I did my homework and studied hard. That was not always popular. I followed the rules because that was what you do. It was not always popular. I have many memories of being the last one picked for paired or group activities. When you don't have long standing friendships, when it comes to working in pairs, it is very difficult. I was always left with the girl who did not want to be in class, or the person who was even less popular than me. I partnered one girl who was not popular, she did not speak very good English and her idea of working in pairs was to get me to do the work for her. I did that for a while, but then another girl had moved into the school, so I got to partner with her for a while until she made friendships of her own. If teachers considered organising the pairings randomly, or rotating groups, things might have been easier for kids like me. I do wonder if it is easier for young people with AS now, perhaps teaching methods have moved on so that the unpopular children are not exposed regularly as always being the odd one out or the last to be picked. Collaborative working is very difficult for someone with AS. I found I was more at ease in classes where the desks were arranged in lines facing the front. I found group work very difficult. Tables arranged in huddles made it more difficult to cope as you also had to listen to other groups around you discussing the task. I find tuning out noise very difficult so I am sure I did not follow all that was said in many of the group activities.

I was terrible at PE, I was picked last for team games. Being a fat kid, wearing glasses and with a bad hair cut was not good for street cred, but also being very uncoordinated and clumsy at PE meant I heard things like "we had her last week, its your turn!" My school report was usually good, but the PE teacher always wrote "could try harder!" did she not realise just how hard I did try? It is hard to make yourself good at sport if you are not very coordinated at team games. I also found the concept of team games difficult. I did not understand who to pass the ball to in netball. If you threw it to the girl who shouted loudest, sometimes the teacher would tell you off, but then if you threw it to the person near the teacher, that was wrong too. Once I got the idea that you found the person who was free of a marker then threw to them, that made it easier, but I found it very challenging, I did not seem to grasp the techniques or concepts as quickly as others. Determined to overcome my past, I even tried playing adult netball with some girls from work, but I only lasted 2 training sessions as I got shouted at so much by the others, I thought I must be a really bad player. Because I was tall I was always put in defence, but when the score was 18 – 0 against us and I was goal defence, I felt the pressure was on me and I felt I let the side down!

The feeling of letting people down was something I felt often. When you believe the things people say and take things literally, then words sometimes even spoken in jest can be very hurtful. Having felt hurt by words so many times, I make it a point not to say things which belittle another person – even if intended as humour. I do take words literally and if someone says something, I think they mean it. I do not find it easy to appreciate that other peoples feelings and interests change and they do not always mean the words that they say. I found teenage innuendos difficult. If someone says "do not chase me" and then they look round expecting you to chase them, I find it confusing. I know my son has similar difficulties with this. He listens to girls say that a boy annoys them because they did something such as put worms in their bag but then the same girl actually likes the boy and does want to be near him. My son finds this very confusing. I enjoy watching "Friends" on video as it shows group friendships and dynamics. I find it interesting as the friends do and say things to each other which could be hurtful and you would expect them to fall out with each other, but they always seem to forgive and move on. Then in the next episode there is no mention of the previous argument or disagreement. I think such acceptance and tolerance of others is something people on the autistic spectrum have to learn. It does not come automatically. I know I can store up lists of misdemeanours which I feel have been done against me by someone, then I have to consciously forgive that person, dump the wrong doing and move on.

I devised a visual way of doing this for my son. He finds expressing his anger and frustrations difficult. When he comes home from school he often has frustrations and anger which he finds hard to express. I have a work sheet which we complete together on the computer. It contains questions which you complete to state why you were angry, what happened, and what you could do about it. My son types in the answers, prints out the sheet, folds it, and then posts it in a shoe box with a slot in the lid. He never takes the sheets out to reread them. It is as if, moment of anger has been expressed, posted and then he can move on.

THE 'Q' FACTOR

People with AS sometimes find it difficult to understand humour or teasing. Taking words literally can make it difficult to shrug off some comments. My son has difficulty at school because one pupil says she is going to kill him. He believes her, and he is terrified of her. My husband has learned not to say "I'm going to kill that dog" or "we have to get rid of that dog" when she eats something she should not as such comments give my son such worries. We also try not to say "we'll never get a parking space!" It will also be taken too literally!

Taking words literally is common to many people on the autistic spectrum, I have written more about this in a later section of this book.

I look back at my childhood and know I was not happy and felt that I did not fit in. I was not sure why; maybe I misinterpreted situations or got things wrong socially. Maybe I spoke too much about my favourite subjects, or maybe I did not understand the implied meanings of what people were saying. Maybe I took things too literally or was too honest; telling someone "yes your bum does look big in that" or "no I do not like your new hairstyle" does not help maintain friendships. I think I lost one friend because I tried to ask too much about her home life. She told me what her mum had bought her for Christmas, so I asked what her dad bought her; I was puzzled why she only said things were from her mum. I did not have the understanding to reason that her mum was a single parent. It must have been painful for my friend to have to explain why her dad did not live with her mum, other girls of 16 would probably have picked up the implied meaning and not pushed for more information. Once I have made such a mistake however, I do try and learn from it and not repeat it, so I am more careful now when talking to someone, but I am sure I still get things wrong.

There were times at school that I did not know why I was singled out and teased or ridiculed. Perhaps I was just the easiest target. Sometimes it was due to my size. In science lessons we had to sit on very uncomfortable stools. I sat in the 3rd row from the front with some other girls but the girls who sat in the back row would laugh about the size of my bottom. I used to sit right back on the stool and perch my legs on the bottom rung, that was the most comfortable position I could find on the stool. Anxious to try and stop the ridiculing I looked at how the other girls sat and realised they perched nearer the front. I found that was very uncomfortable, but to try and stop the giggling and pointing behind me I used to sit as far forward as I could and keep my feet on the floor lifting my behind as much as I could so it looked smaller, or I used to sit to one side so that I leaned on one side of my backside only. I had back and leg ache but it did stop the ridicule.

At school, I was so unhappy in one class at school that my parents requested that I be moved into a

THE 'Q' FACTOR

different class. I was so badly bullied; I was called "4 eyes" and "boff", and all the usual names for someone who isn't popular. There were times when I knew why I was being targeted and made fun of, but sometimes I did not even understand what they were teasing me about. They were laughing, at me, but I could not understand why.

Moving class did make it easier as there were many girls in the new class who were interested in music, so I had a peer group for the first time. The form teacher was the music teacher, and he was very kind. He gave me jobs to do and showed faith in me so I did get some confidence back. The girls in the class did include me, but I was different. I must have been difficult to get along with and I drifted in the class trying to find a good friend. I was desperate to fit in and wanted to be popular, but I did not know how.

I was not interested in fashion until I was 17 – even when I tried to follow fashion, I did not always get it right. I would often start wearing something just as it was on the way out; I was still wearing wedge shoes a remnant of the late 70s long after the pixie boots and stilettos with bows came in during the 80s. I did not wear make up until 6th form and I was still wearing knee length socks until 17. I only stopped wearing them because a friend asked me if was going to carry on wearing knee length socks all my life!

This girl was someone who I thought of as a very good friend, but on reflection, she often used me as a target for humiliation. She liked to tease me as I was a fat kid, she seemed happy to make fun of me. We were both involved in the local guides for a few years, as older girls we helped out and one year she wrote a play for the Christmas show. I was in the play, but my friend was happy to direct. Instead of directing on the night of the performance, she sat in the audience and laughed at my humiliation as no one was organising the young girls back stage and prompting them or directing them to be in the right place at the right time. I was on stage as Widow Twanky saying the cue line for the next actor to come on, but no one came on. I can follow a script, but "ad lib" is not one of my strengths, so I was mortified that I stood on the stage for a number of minutes and eventually, I had to go back stage and pull the girl forward from the back of the gang of young guides all watching behind the scenes and but not concentrating on their own entrances or exits. They were only 11 years old, I don't blame them at all, but this incident showed my friendship for what it was.

This is an example of how easily a person with AS can be manipulated and made the object of fun. I took the performance seriously, but my friend more sophisticated and mature than I understood that it was probably going to be a disaster and she preferred to distance herself from it and enjoyed watching my humiliation. She sat with the parents

THE 'Q' FACTOR

and shared their laughter as they all enjoyed watching the poorly acted and choreographed play. I felt hurt by her actions, we had spent hours rehearsing the enthusiastic young guides and I thought we would manage to put on a good play. It was a lesson for me that I although I liked directing others, I am not really very good at it.

4th year options made things at school easier for me, as the class groupings were changed as you chose subjects and the classes were streamed according to ability. This meant I was not in the same group as many of the girls who bullied me. Because I worked hard I was in the top groups for my subjects. It was a struggle in maths as I do not find the subject easy, but my Dad and brother tutored me at home and coached me through the work, so I scraped a pass at GCE.

I did not find learning difficult as in my teens the curriculum was fact based, I found it easy to learn and retain facts. I could relate the entire periodic table in chemistry and read the entire diagram of the alimentary canal from pictures in my head, but I found applying the information and concepts difficult. I found the structure of exams suited me, you learn the facts, go into a room in quiet, sit at a designated desk so there was no fear of being left out or not knowing where to sit. You read the exam paper; followed instructions then went ahead and did it. I learnt a big lesson at primary school bout reading the entire exam paper right through before you start. In the last year at primary school we had a series of tests including the 11+ exam. I was not sure which particular test it was, but my teacher verbally told us at the beginning to read the test paper through first. I was one of the many pupils who were caught out and did not read the entire list of questions. I did as I was told and remember reading the first page, but did not turn over and read the second page. I could see people around me writing and I was worried that I would not have enough time. So I too started answering the questions. We all worked through the test paper and then the last question said "only answer question 40." I think only 1 boy did the paper correctly.

After that lesson, I always read exams or questions first; I also apply the same approach to application forms and questionnaires. It is helpful to read the entire form or exam through as you can see what is expected of your answers. I might interpret one question a certain way, but then I read on and see that a later question actually covers what I thought I should answer initially, so I revise my answer and read on.

I found I was best at multiple choice questions and at GCE level each subject had a multiple choice paper in the exams. I found essay writing difficult, I would write what I thought was my best ever attempt and the teacher would mark it as B- or B at best. Perhaps my difficulty was interpreting the questions. My highest grades were in biology which was all about learning facts and I wrote pages in my exam. My lowest grade was in English literature, I did not find analysing poetry easy, but I was good at memorising quotes, so I put as many of them into the essays as I could. I failed my German O level, I do not understand why. All but one girl in the class failed; perhaps that was a reflection more on the teaching than the pupils. I got 100% in my computer science final exam; the teacher told me he even marked the paper several times as he had never had a pupil attain that mark previously. I found the computer science syllabus easy as it is logical.

So, I did not have the happiest childhood. In an attempt to fit in and be more popular, I went on a diet. The final straw after years of teasing about being fat was when a so called friend teased me badly about needing an extra large lab coat for chemistry, so I decided to lose weight. It took me 2 years but I went from a size 18 to a size 10. I must have been very difficult to live with during that time as I know I get grumpy when I am hungry. And following a diet I was constantly hungry. As one of the strengths of AS is following rules and structure, I found it easy to follow the rules of a diet but as another characteristic of AS is the tendency to fixate on things, I became too fixated on losing the weight and I developed an eating disorder I have since struggled with for many years.

I am not saying that I developed an eating disorder because I had undiagnosed AS, but I have read that it is common in teenagers with undiagnosed AS. There is a desire to have control in your life, and food can become the focus. People with AS can be very determined, and find self discipline easy. Following rules is easy, so once I decided to count the calories and not exceed 1500 each day, I found that easy. It became obsessive and did not know when to stop counting the calories. I made myself eat fewer and fewer calories until I was only eating about 500 calories a day. I believed losing weight would improve my popularity. I did get compliments when I was smaller in size, so I carried on dieting.

So I have admitted that I have had difficulty with eating disorders, because the counting calories did lead to binge eating too, which then lead to purging in a desperate attempt to stay thin.

I do not understand the psychology and why eating disorders can take hold and become so difficult to overcome, but I am now a happier rounded size 14 who does not count calories. I do not even know what I weigh.

I have also struggled with depression, this started in my teens. I was frequently frustrated and angry and found it difficult to express my feelings and even understand why I felt the way I did. I found it very difficult to talk about the way I felt, so I withdrew and spent time on my own. I have since read that depression is anger turned inwards. I can express anger, but it usually comes out as an explosion following hours or days of holding the feelings inside. When I reach an overload of feelings and frustrations, there is usually a small trigger which might even be unrelated to the main cause. But then I do literally see red in my head, I lose sight of all thought and pictures; I cannot read any diagrams or lists or the dictionary in my head. I then erupt in anger. I usually feel very bad about the outbursts and do not like that about myself.

As a teenager, although my close family might disagree, I used to try to keep my frustrations inside and let of steam in the privacy of my bedroom. I would talk to myself and voice some of the frustrations while I was alone. There always seemed to be more anger than I could voice, so I was left feeling frustrated. I could not find a way to express the feelings and then move on. I know I was a very volatile child and I was told that I had a bad temper. Family members used to describe me as "prickly" or cross. I think I found the school day so difficult, trying to conform, fit in and understand things around me that I had many frustrations and confusions which I could not express or speak about.

As an adult, I now ask about things I do not understand. I ask my husband why people react the way they do, or what has upset them or made them behave in a certain way. Sometimes however, I am embarrassed to admit that I do not understand, so I silently sit and wonder, but do not really seem to comprehend what is going on around me.

I think I internalise a lot and think carefully about situations and what people say. I get the impression that other people do not ponder on information in the same way. They seem more "happy go lucky" and less burdened by the desire to understand and fit in.

The feeling of isolation and difficulties understanding other people often overwhelms me. I feel sad that I do not understand people very well and sad that I am not very good company. At school sports day, I am the person sitting alone on the bench; other parents group together or arrive together and seem to enjoy each others company. I am happy to sit alone, but I am aware that it might look odd. Children are very good at filling the gaps; my daughter will come over and bring her friend too. Then the friend's parent will come and sit down and we can discuss how the children have done in their races and hope we can get away with not running the mothers race again for another year!

As I have struggled with depression, I have been prescribed anti depressants which I have taken on and off over the years. I am now happy with the medication I am taking as it helps my anxiety levels. It was initially prescribed to help with pain relief, but as a side effect I do not feel so edgy or so much anxiety or frustration all the time. I still

THE 'Q' FACTOR

find social occasions very difficult, but I do not
have the same level of internal anxiety and stress.

ME

Common to many people with AS I find social situations and new situations difficult. My heart beat would race and I get dry mouth and sweaty palms. The adrenaline must have been racing through my body on a daily basis.

I developed Myalargic encephalitis in 2003. It crept up on me but I think having ME has actually curbed some of the AS obsessions I have had in my life. I believe the ME crept into my body due to the prolonged stress I was under. Living with anyone on the autistic spectrum is challenging and brings a degree of stress into your life. I was living with 2 sons who were unhappy at the time I developed ME, and I was struggling with my own obsessions and anxieties. I was trying to juggle working, doing too much voluntary work, on too many committees, training for a marathon, training a puppy, rehearsing for a local drama festival play, and fitting into a new community. My health gave way and I became unwell. I did also have a severe viral infection but I carried on as normal and trained through it. I was following a marathon training regime for the London marathon which was designed by Roger Black. It was a very good training programme, but I should have stopped the training while I was unwell. I did not. The training programme became an obsession, I had to follow it without fail or I believed I would not manage the marathon. I felt the symptoms creep into my life, but ignored them until the point of collapse at work.

Having AS does make it difficult to relate to how your body feels and it makes it difficult to describe how the symptoms feel. I find it very difficult to explain when asked to describe pain. Does it feel a burning pain, stabbing pain or throbbing pain, I find that very difficult. I can tune out pain until it becomes too severe, and then I find I cannot block it out at all. I know I must have a fairly high pain threshold as when I went on my training runs I would feel pain in my feet, but my determination to follow the training regime meant I carried on. I push myself through any pain using the breathing technique they teach in antenatal classes. I concentrate of the pattern of breathing in and out and it does take the focus off the pain. When I got home after one such training run, I found I had lost 3 toe nails and had blisters which were bleeding badly. I could shut out the pain by focusing on the running and my breathing technique. One step at a time, breathing in and out, one lamp post at a time, patterns of dotted white lines on the road until I got the distance done.

Having ME brought brain fog, this totally took over and that was the main thing I struggled with for many months. I had memory difficulties, so I could not rely on my memory any more. I have always had a very good memory, when working as a Personnel Manager I could rattle off the entire staff dates of birth and National insurance numbers and home phone numbers, but at my worst with ME, I could not even remember my Dads birthday. I knew it was in May but I could not remember if it was 26th, 27th or 29th. I didn't want to admit to my parents that I could not remember, so I used to send a card in advance of the 3 dates. Sometimes I would phone my Mum and try and find out what date it was by asking her what plans she had for "the special day" hoping I might get a clue. If she said "oh well on Tuesday of course we will be going out for a meal, but at the weekend we will be having a bit of a get together too." Then I would know the date.

As well as the memory difficulties and brain fog, the physical symptoms of ME were also hard for me. I am so used to driving myself and pushing myself to the limit so suddenly having to admit that I could not walk up a flight of stairs without help was very difficult. I had severe pain in my arms and legs most of the time and swollen glands in my neck. I was fatigued beyond tired, I had no strength in my muscles. I had not even got the energy to finish a sentence and I could not coordinate my arms and legs very well any more.

Is ME a mental health condition? I do not know but there is research and evidence to suggest that it can be caused or triggered by a virus. Did I develop the ME because I had undiagnosed AS? I do not know, but having the ME gave me time to think, time to read and time to consider.

THE 'Q' FACTOR

I read many books about Autism, and it revealed so much to me about my own life, that I started my journey to diagnosis. The ME stripped me of some of the strategies I had developed to cope with the difficulties my AS brings. I had relied on memory to cope with difficulty in processing and decoding information. Due to the brain fog, I could not read the encyclopaedia or pictures in my head. So I could not decode abbreviations as easily and I found it more difficult to remember things. I would lose my place in conversations and forget the plot on TV programmes or reading books. I sometimes forget fingerings for my musical instruments; things I have known for 30 years, I forget things which should be totally embedded into my personality.

I became slower of thinking, and I started to understand that I had been using my memory and ability to see things visually to help me understand things. For example, I would use a visual memory of a meeting to recall who sat where, their role within the group and how the meeting would run. The visual memory would prompt me to recall the discussions at previous meetings, who led the discussions, the etiquette of the group and what was expected of me. Without my memory, I would feel confusion and more anxiety. Each meeting would feel like a totally new situation again and I would have trouble bringing my thought process into line with the type of meeting, recalling the jargon, the direction the group was going and the way the discussions took place. When the brain fog lifted as I recovered from ME, I could read the pictures again. The pictures would be images of the information necessary for the meeting, of the minutes or reports I had read, and I could hear the conversations in my head and recall the discussions and decisions made previously.

I think having the ME has given me greater understanding into AS. Abilities I took for granted became a challenge. I was compensating for some areas of difficulty with understanding and decoding situations by relying on memory. When meeting someone I have a stock list of questions in my head to keep the conversation going. I ask if the person has holiday plans and how the family are doing. I used to remember conversations I had with people very easily and my husband and boss used to say I had a phenomenal memory, now I find I cannot even remember why I am arguing with my husband. We laugh, as I have to admit "I cannot remember what I am arguing with you about, but I know I am upset with you about something!" Perhaps ME has saved my marriage!

I think having undiagnosed AS is more difficult to cope with than the actual "label." For me diagnosis has really helped me understand so many things I have found difficult in my life. I find it much easier to accept myself now as "different" rather than being stupid or inferior or odd.
I have wondered when to talk to my son about being different. He has had many times when he has cried about feeling different. He asks why he

THE 'Q' FACTOR

finds it so hard to understand things. He gets very angry with himself if he doesn't understand something. It reminds me so much of myself. He asks why he always needs someone to help him, why does he need a carer and his sister doesn't? However, he does actually really enjoy having 1-1 attention from a carer and so after much discussion about it, we can now use this as one of the positives about being different.

I have been told that the earlier you tell your child the better it is, but having only learnt this about myself at 41, I do feel that there is no time pressure. It doesn't actually change anything or provide a cure. It is just a way of finding self acceptance and understanding. We have sat down with my son on many occasions and talked about being different, but he finds it very difficult to understand the concept.

When I was asked to do a talk on being a parent of a child with Autism, I was preparing some slides and I asked my son permission to use some photographs and to speak about him. I was worried about hurting his feelings. He asked me "is that because of autism?" and I just said yes, he was quite happy and walked away!

Routine

You have to mention this when writing about autism or Aspergers Syndrome.

I think I could make this shorter and just say, routine is **very** important to Ben! It is also very important to me, as people with AS like routine.

At home we use visual timetables, check lists, timers, toy clocks to get through the day. I refer to a calendar and diary each day for my own activities and for my children.

What do parents do the night before a school holiday? I am unusually up late on the computer preparing a timetable of the weeks of the holiday and breaking down each day into segments of time. This is printed, laminated and displayed on our kitchen door.

Visual timetables and social stories are excellent tools for living with autism they are fantastic. We can get through the worst change and disruptions if we plan ahead, use a visual timetable and social stories. We use lots of repetition, answer the same questions over and over, refer to the timetables and calendar.

I use one specifically for any thing out of the ordinary, that can be anything from Christmas, birthdays, Lauren having a friend to play, me

THE 'Q' FACTOR

having a music rehearsal, going to the doctor or dentist etc.

Some sections of the timetable I can leave blank or call "time to play" as now at 15 my son does like an element of choice, but mostly I have to allocate the chunks of the day.

I have also learnt to have a "wild card" I call it that, but my son knows it as "change of activity" taking language literally is another characteristic of autism and I think if I said we are going to use our wild card now, my son would imagine a card which might contain a real tiger or crocodile. It would be a dangerous chart to use and certainly not make my day any easier!

I notice friends now visit and always check the kitchen door to see what timetables or sticker charts we are working on!

Routine and normality are very important. Disruptions to this can cause anxiety and I do think that with so much going on around our children at school and in the world, some normality and routine is essential and comforting. Coping at school is exhausting and draining, there are changes to routines all the time, so trying to maintain normality at home helps minimise the stress and anxiety.

When my husband finally persuaded me to let him decorate our kitchen, for his peace of mind, the sake of our marriage and his relationship with Ben, I took myself and the kids south to stay with granny for a two week holiday. The disruption to routine would been so difficult for me personally and also for the children. Sadly the time was not quite long enough as we all know with home improvements, you start something and you find another difficulty and it slows things down.

Malcolm used a computer programme to plan the layout of the kitchen, so I had a visual picture of what it would be like. This helped me adapt to the idea of the changes. When we got home, it was amazing, the room was transformed, a wall removed so we had a kitchen diner, new cupboards, lovely white walls but due to things not being delivered on time and hold ups, no carpet and no lighting. My husband was using a room downstairs as a kitchen the contents were still boxed in the living room. The dining table was flat packed and chairs stacked to one side.

Malc asked what we thought, I honestly said, I love it.
Ben's words were very memorable:
"will I *ever* be able to eat my dinner at the table ever again!"
I think if the room had nothing else in it, if the table had been up with the chairs around it and Ben's place mat there for him it would have been perfect.

THE 'Q' FACTOR

I had lovely new cupboard space, lots more room, but I still had to put things in the places where Ben could find them. So his marmite, vitamin tablets and night time medication were all put in the same place as before.

I try and encourage Ben doing some things for himself, so I had to put cups and plates in the same spot as before, I found if I tried to move things, he would always put them back in their old spot anyway so it was just confusing for everyone else.

Routine is so important to people with autism, even on Christmas morning, much to Laurens dismay, Ben has to get up watch lazy town at 7am, have his hot chocolate and then a bath, get dressed and then prepare for breakfast.

After breakfast, we can start the festivities. Then we start the Christmas day routine, we have to do things the same as other years. Ben likes to get the presents from under the tree and distribute them in a loud voice reading the labels accordingly. It becomes difficult when he can't read Great Aunty Barbara's writing, and what on earth is supposed to happen with joint presents!

I always feel under pressure about Christmas, Ben writes his Christmas list in early summer, usually July, and adds to it right up to Christmas morning! This year he presented me with a long list of his favourite model trains - DMUs, (Diesel Multiple

Units) with specific and detailed information about each one. I got him to show me his top 3 DMUs and then with the wonder of the WWW (World Wide Web) we got one in time! I have to be very careful on the computer, not to leave a trace of the sites I have looked at. I even get phone calls from school, it is Ben to tell me the thing I am bidding on Ebay, well I have just been outbid! I got a good friend to help me out and bid for me and we got the yellow hair mermaid he really wanted so his Christmas was okay! Phew!

At night we have set routine. Ben gets ready for bed independently now once he has been prised away from his computer, he will get himself ready with just a few prompts which is great, but what ever you are doing, you have to brace yourself for the 9.12 tuck in! I hope I have remembered to make up his bed if it had to be changed, or else that has to be done immediately. Ben comes down to find me where ever I am with an arm full of soft toys. I have to acknowledge each toy, flick them with my finger and then say prayers. I cannot leave it there, I must check his teeth and say "good teeth cleaning, off to bed, sleep well" then I hope I can return to the tv programme I am missing or carry on the music rehearsal with a room full of patient friends who all kindly say "good night Ben"

Once we have done that routine, then Ben will usually go to bed, but I have to follow a little and prevent Ben from harassing which ever pet is in range and see him into his room. He is easily distracted and when passing the music room for example, he might remember he should have played his violin, so he will go in and do that and then the tuck in routine starts all over again. You cannot skip stages, or rush him at all, if you try, he gets flustered and more difficult to manage.

Once in bed, it is peaceful until 6am.

Holidays are sometimes difficult when Ben tries to stick to his routine. We were helping at a youth camp last summer and Ben stuck to his routine. The rest of the youngsters were busy involved in an activity but at 9pm Ben strode in pyjamas, with an arm full of pink furry teddy bears in pyjamas and slippers waiting for me to do his night time tuck in routine!

The London Marathon

In 2002 I ran the London Marathon. I started running when Ben was 3. I got fitter as he was so active and an escaper, I spent a lot of time running after him. His early years were a bit stressful too – especially around the time of his diagnosis. I found running and exercise helped me cope with the stress. After a day of meetings and receiving Ben's diagnosis, I went to the gym and pounded 20 minutes on the treadmill. I was so focused on what I was doing; I did not notice people around me were watching. When I finished, a lady asked me if I competed in running events, I laughed and told her I could not run, I was always last at school. She told me I should join a running club and maybe run a ½ marathon; I thought I probably couldn't run that far. It made me think however and I did continue the running. I started gradually lengthening the distance to see if I could do it. Then I entered a local ½ marathon. I got hooked on running, but decided I did not like long distances. I did 3 miles most days and that distance suited me. It is a great way to get out on your own and get some exercise. It was the time of day when I put my brain into neutral. I didn't think much beyond the next lamppost, no one put pressure on me as I ran, I didn't have to conform or worry about getting it wrong as I was on my own and at my own pace.

Running became part of my routine. I would not feel happy about my day unless I got to go running

THE 'Q' FACTOR

either first thing in the morning or at lunch time at the gym at work. I had to get up very early to fit a morning run in, but it used to work around our schedule at home. I would run at 6.45 for 25 minutes, I could do a 3 mile route in that time. Then I would shower and get Ben ready. Meanwhile Malcolm would get himself ready and oversee the children before starting his journey with Nick and Lauren to my parents house to drop them off for school. Nick was independent enough to get his own breakfast and he got himself ready for school. Lauren would probably be unfed or eat her toast in the car and still in her pyjamas but by 7.30 they would be on their way and I would be ready for work and could get Ben ready for his taxi pick up at 8am. I would be at the car ready to strap him into the taxi and then at 8.03 I would be off on my journey to work too.

I did enter the London marathon a few times, but didn't get accepted until I had moved to Orkney! I thought it was ironic that I moved away from London in the August and then following April I was back in London running the marathon.

When I got the acceptance letter, I was stunned. I had entered for the 5th time thinking I would not get a place. Perhaps being nearer 40 and also estimating a finishing time of over 5 hours combined with a postcode in the North islands, got me picked.

The acceptance pack included the training schedule written by Roger Black. I stuck to that schedule rigidly. The marathon became my obsession. I spoke about it all the time; I read everything I could find about marathon training. I got advice from other runners. I bought the kit for the job. I would not run in anything other than flat lock seam running leggings. I had learnt the hard way that bulgy seams could cause blisters in very painful places! I wore the brand of running shoes which were reputed to be the best. I was even selective about which socks I wore. I bought the biggest tub of Vaseline I could find and systematically smeared my feet and ankles before each run. I rigidly stuck to the running magazine recommended rules. I ate carbohydrate 30 minutes before each run, drank the recommended fluids. I was really focused in my approach.

Part of my motivation was to help raise funds for a new mini bus for my son's school. There were only 16 pupils in the school and all the parents were busy caring for their child. This meant that there were few families to help with fundraising. The school needed a new minibus as their current one was not suitable for some of the children's wheelchairs. Some of the children had health conditions which mean the parents were very busy with caring responsibilities. The fundraising really motivated me.

I watched a film "Clockwork Mice." It is about a teacher who works in a school for children who are disaffected with school and family life, their behaviour was very challenging. In the film, the teacher encourages the pupils to take up running. His running club involved even the most disaffected. He told the pupils "I run because I like it I run because I can."

The faces of the children at my son's school motivated me to keep running. The words "because I can" meant a great deal. Many of the children at the school were not able to attempt such a run without physical support, equipment, carers and much motivation. The faces of some the children speak of their daily achievements as difficult as any marathon. To many of them, life's daily struggles are difficult and physically hard to bear. Their families know the strife and hardship endured by the children locked inside their additional support needs.

Running into strong Orkney wind and rain, up hill, through snow or ice, when I was physically tired during a long hard run, I would ask myself "why am I doing this?" I focused on the faces and smiles of the children and reminded myself "I run because I like it, I run because I can."

I think having AS made it easier training for a huge event such as the marathon. I was very single minded about training, fatigue or ill health didn't deter me from my training schedule. The training dominated my life for 6 months. I didn't question the training schedule or cheat in any way, I followed it rigidly. While training I changed my diet and eating patterns. During the month before the event, I concentrated on carb loading. You eat more carbohydrates so that you build up stores for the event. It was a good excuse to eat more cakes so I enjoyed that element to the training. I could eat what I liked and did not put on any weight. My body shape changed as I was running up to 60 miles a week in the last month before the big day.

Morse my golden retriever dog used to be my training companion, but the time came when I had to leave him behind. The distances got too long and he was too slow, so I stopped taking him running. He was very sad to be left behind and got a bit over weight without the exercise, but I made the decision because the last time I took him, he was so slow and pulled me back. He wouldn't run on the lead on the verge, it was okay when he was off lead as he bumbled about but always caught me up at the right time. Once we had to run on roads to do the required distance, he could not be off lead but he hated running on the grass verge, and insisted on running on the tarmac behind me. I had gone 2 miles but still had 4 to do. I decided to tie Morse to a fence post safely out of danger of the road and continue without him. I was doing a there and back route, so I would collect him on the way back. I ran on, but couldn't help worry that he might be in trouble. I thought someone might see him, think he was abandoned and take him away. I also worried that he would slip his collar and end

THE 'Q' FACTOR

up in the field with livestock and get shot. So I
think that was the fastest 2 miles I had ever run
before I colleted him and then took him the final 2
miles home again. After that run, Morse got left at
home.

As I've written earlier in this book, I was foolish
and I trained through a viral infection. I was
feeling quite unwell and had very little energy, but
I forced myself out into the January weather and
continued. I think I only missed 1 or 2 training
runs during in the whole programme. I had the
schedule stuck on the kitchen door and ticked off
each run. The only variation I made to the
programme was to make my long run on a
Saturday instead of the Sunday. I can remember
being very frustrated by the weather. We had
snow for a few days and the icy conditions made
road running very treacherous. I found it difficult
to find a route which was safe enough to use for
any long distance, so I used to run back wards
and forwards up and down the hill where I live for
the same amount of time I would usually run the
required distance on the training schedule. I
figured I might not be doing the exact mileage, but
the length time was right. It was actually very
tough as the hill is very steep, but the snow
banked up on the edges of the main roads meant
it was too dangerous to run on any other roads
nearby. Orkney drivers are very considerate and
always allow runners or cyclists room on the road,
but snow makes even Orkney drivers struggle to
manoeuvre safely out of the way of a runner. My

feet got wet and cold in the ice and snow, but determination drove me to continue.

I forbade myself to use a treadmill in the gym as it is so much easier than road running. I knew I had to get my miles done on the road. I only turned back on a run once. That was when there was snow on the ground but what made the going too difficult was the wind was gusting at 70 miles per hour. I found my running jacket inflated like a sail and I was being gagged by it around my neck. I could not make any momentum in that wind and I turned back after only completing 18 miles of my 22 mile distance. I was gutted. I ran back to the leisure centre in Kirkwall and phoned my husband from there. He came to collect me, but he knows that I was upset not to have made my target on the training schedule that day.

It was foolish not to listen to the limits of my body. That is something that people on the autistic spectrum find very difficult. The determination and focus keeps you going. When fixated on something, you might forget to eat, or actually not associate the hunger pangs with the need to eat, the obsession drives you on. I did pay a price for training through the illness, as after the marathon I didn't really get my energy levels back. I started getting the symptoms of ME, but at the time of the marathon, I was so determined that even losing toe nails or blisters in places where you do not want to imagine, I continued regardless.

THE 'Q' FACTOR

What helped me complete the training was breaking it down into manageable chunks. I was used to helping my son do that with difficult talks so I used that approach with my running. On a very long distance I just focused on the next fence post and kept moving forward literally thinking about one step at a time. If I looked ahead at months on the training schedule and saw the length of running time increasing, I felt overwhelmed, so I chose to only focus on the week I was doing. I seldom thought about the whole 26 miles. I was a bit fazed by the map of the marathon route which I received 2 days before the event. That was the first time I really considered the distance as a whole. Previously I had only thought about it as mile after mile and only in relation to my longest run up to that date.

On the day of the event I do not remember the land marks along the route. I concentrated on my feet – determined not to trip on one of the discarded water bottles. I do remember going over Tower Bridge, but later when I saw the coverage on TV, I was surprised that I managed to run past the Tower of London without noticing it! I think that shows how single minded and focused someone with AS can get, determination and focus pushing you on. I managed a good time

I am glad that I did the London Marathon, it is a memory I will always have. I am now content to watch it on TV! I do wish I could do things without being quite so obsessed or focused. It doesn't seem very easy for me to be half hearted about something. I suspect people living with someone on the autistic spectrum wish that we could be less obsessed about things too!

The collector!

I don't think my son Ben is unique in that he loves to collect things, but, this is collecting with a difference. If he gets one soft toy, he likes to collect the set. We had trouble getting the 1 jelly cat mermaid to complete the collection of 4! I am of the opinion that toy manufacturers must have done research into the desire to collect things as different toys come in not only different colours, but the whole set is also available in pocket size or in large size and there is also the ultimate battery operated version, so for example we had a collection of teletubbies, we had 4 hard plastic ones, 4 beanie ones, 4 beanie ones with key ring attachment, 4 large size and 1 battery operated laa laa – the ultimate prize for Ben after he survived an operation in hospital – but that is another chapter!

My son Nick is a collector, at the age of 17 was still adding to a boglin collection he started at 5 years old. He collected the football stickers or what ever play ground faze was around, but after other children have got bored with it and moved on, the collector still keeps going.

The collection becomes a focus and obsession. They must have whatever it is they need to complete it and it dominates thought and conversation. It becomes expensive and annoying and often the collection is not something other children collect. The pokemon cards were a classic example, we still have them lovingly stored in albums. Nick knows the current values of each card! The collection can be a real motivating factor for learning and retaining facts. It's amazing how a child can reel off the facts and figures of an entire series of animation cards or stickers, but forget to tell you that they have cooking tomorrow and they need a bag of icing sugar which you don't happen to have and the shops have shut!

When I was a child, I had a fascination for stag beetles. I think it was a solitary interest. I collected them. I looked at facts in books about them, drew pictures of them, and knew how to pick them up without discomfort to the stage beetle. You had to grab them using your thumb and forefinger on the top and bottom of the abdomen. From behind so they did not pinch you with their claws. If you held them along their legs that could cut off their breathing so I was very careful as I held them. I used to collect them after school and smuggle them into my class the next day and put them in my stag beetle environment. It was an empty desk next to mine and I arranged leaves and grass for them. At play time I could collect new grass, but I don't remember throwing any grass away after it went mouldy, so I think that is why I arrived one morning to find the desk empty. It was probably very unpleasant as I had quite a number in there for some time. I was too upset but worried to speak about it. I was devastated that my stag beetles had gone, but I could not tell anyone as I knew I would get told off. I am sure the teacher

THE 'Q' FACTOR

knew about it, but chose not to punish me. I am
not sure why. I don't think stag beetles are very
common now, I hope my activities did not
contribute to their decline! Now as I reflect on that
memory, I am sure the pungent odour gave my
prized collection away or possibly one of the
prized male stag beetles terrorised the cleaning
lady as she dusted the desk! I thought it quite
normal to collect and study them; I would spend
hours trapping them and reading facts about them
in encyclopaedias. The access to the internet our
children now have must make autistic obsessions
much easier to study.

My obsessions have changed as I have grown up,
which is the same with my boys. I currently bore
people about access issues, playing the bassoon
or training my dog which I love. People ask me
about the dog, but I notice their expression glazes
over, so I know it is time to stop talking about it.
My husband is very long suffering about it, but
even he finds it annoying. My dog is a registered
Therapet visitor which is a voluntary activity which
I love. She had the huge honour of being voted
Therapet of the year in Scotland 2006. This
meant we had to travel to Edinburgh to collect the
award. My husband sighed and said

"oh you and THAT dog!"

It helps if you find an acceptable obsession,
people tend to go along with you and challenge it
less if it is conventional or acceptable. Many boys

can talk about football without much cause for concern, but rattling on about car number plates from regions of England which I used to do was possibly a bit odd.

Food fads

Every child has likes and dislikes, but maybe a child with autism takes this to extreme. I must have a supply of marmite in the house and must carry it with me when we go out, we must have cartons of raisins for pack lunch boxes and we must have Heinz spaghetti hoops! No other brand will do. It doesn't usually occur to children to tell you when they are nearly finished the box of wheetos, they may even put an empty box away after they have had breakfast, but the next day, when faced with the empty box, the consequences of their actions don't matter, the fact is the day is totally ruined and the peace gone because we don't have wheetos for breakfast!

With my son, I would grasp the fad which could be - only *goodfellas* thin and crispy pepperoni pizza, I would buy a stack of supplies and then he would tell me, "I don't like that anymore, I like noodles" the dog does quite well out of this arrangement.

Malcolm now knows well the supplies which are autism folk only! Touch them if you dare,

We try and get Ben to eat more variety of foods, but it is a trial. We can get away with quite a bit if we put gravy on it, but we learnt early that it is better to have peaceful meal times with a compromise on menu than a battle and tantrum which would last hours and solve nothing but make the parents more stressed and the food fad worse anyway.

Hard as it is to admit, I have food fads too. I like brown bread and marmalade for breakfast and I am very fussy about how I take my tea. I cannot stand milky weak tea; it makes me feel physically sick. I do not like eggs and find it very difficult to vary my diet. When I find something I like, I stick to it until I realise I am being very boring and must try and change what I am eating. I go through fads, I will eat cheese toasties for lunch for ages, and suddenly I grow tired of them and move onto something else – but sandwiches are my preferred serving suggestion at lunch time. I find myself drawn to the same foods when I go shopping and my husband is very tolerant, because he must get bored of the monotony.

Despite trying to pretend that I am very easy going about food, I think people close to me know that I am fairly fussy really.

Echolalia

If you don't know what this is it can be a bit weird. Some children with autism repeat what you say, quite literally mimicking tone and intonation. There is immediate echolalia and delayed echolalia. I have read books which state that immediate echolalia is meaningless; however, I believe it had great meaning for the person using it. It is a way of communicating.

Delayed echolalia can be either a way for a person who has difficulty with language joining in a conversation. They might lift a whole phrase or monologue from memory and relate it during a conversation. They might relay the phrase or quote at inappropriate times – which can be a bit annoying!

Ben is an echolalia expert. When he was young, this was his way of communicating. You asked him a question and you just got the same question repeated back to you. It became tricky if you were trying to ask him to choose something. You would say would you like ribena or milk? He would repeat both choices back to you, so you couldn't rely on what he said as his actual choice. I noticed that if someone new was talking to Ben, he would use echolalia but only repeating the last part of the phrase. If they asked him a question giving choices, he might only repeat the last choice, but this didn't necessarily mean that was his preferred option. It was confusing at times.

Ben would also remember conversations he had with people when he only saw them intermittently. He had a wonderful Crossroads Care Attendant who noticed that each time she saw him he would repeat things she had said in previous weeks – word for word. This showed an incredible memory, she might forget the things she had said, but Ben did not. It was almost as if Ben wanted to start a conversation with his friend, but found it difficult to make his own sentences so he would use his carer's exact phrases as this always brought a smile and more conversation. When it was bed time, he would say "where's hedgepig" (this was the word his Care Attendant used for one of his soft toys). Ben knew that saying this would mean stories and soft toys and bed time.

Echolalia could also be used to fill in silence or as narration for a game. Ben would repeat the Thomas the tank engine stories word for word as he heard them on his videos. He would lie on the floor watching the wheels of his trains and say the words of the stories.

I think echolalia is the beginning of learning language; most small children copy what you say, and gradually take the words and use them for themselves. People who use echolalia are communicating and learning language, I think it exemplifies some of the strengths of people with autism – the ability to observe with attention to detail, incredible memory and exceptional auditory skills.

 It can be taken as rudeness if you say something to a child and they repeat what you say – as a toddler that is acceptable, but as an older child this could be assumed as rudeness. Ben is an excellent mimic, and still copies sounds he finds interesting. This might be mobile phone ring tones, some people's laughter or coughing, sounds made by animals, airport announcements – the list goes on. This can be funny or really annoying. Ben repeats songs and dialogue from his favourite films. It is almost as if it helps him internalise the words and understand better. Echolalia is okay if people understand what it is. It is embarrassing in a quiet moment in church for example when Ben pipes up copying something he finds interesting, either a comment whispered by a person sitting near by or something the minister says.

He also likes to repeat chunks of dialogue at inappropriate times, something triggers a memory and he can rattle off whole speeches from a film or from a book. I have found that sshhh doesn't work, neither does my hard stare, I usually have to engage with him, taking the part of a character and ending his monologue by talking as if I am his favourite character giving him the command. Or I side track him by writing something fast about his favourite subject trains.

Sometimes I still use sign language which Ben learnt at his first primary school in England. He still knows the sign language for "enough"! That will usually be enough to trigger some silly signing which is at least quiet so not quite as distracting as the echolalia. When Ben descends into uncontrollable laughter at his own jokes however, nothing will silence him. His laugh is infectious and you usually don't want to stop this at all, but it might at a time when it is not appropriate.

Until the age of 6 Ben could not make some sounds at all. Due to a congenital short soft sub mucal palette He could not say F, V, and food used to get stuck in his throat. He had an operation at great Ormond Street to repair the palette and although a very stressful week for us, it worked and the result was amazing. I almost crashed the car when Ben said to me
"that's a lovely van over there"
It would have previously been
"fats a lubberly fvpan oder dere

With echolalia there might also be copying of mannerisms. This can be embarrassing when you are out and Ben mimics someone in a public place. Airports are the worst as you see lots of people, Ben coughed and sneezed after someone sitting in the waiting area, it was very embarrassing as it was so obvious he was mimicking them.

THE 'Q' FACTOR

I have noticed that Ben still uses echolalia at
social gatherings when he finds it difficult to join in
a conversation. If people are talking in groups
after a church service, Ben will hover behind
someone he knows and mimic them quite loudly. It
is okay if they understand it is his way of trying to
join in or get attention, but it can be taken as
rudeness. He might also stand near a person he
knows and focus on someone else who is a
distance away, copying them and using echolalia.
This means I cannot usually have an uninterrupted
conversation myself as I am constantly aware of
Ben and trying to ensure he doesn't offend
someone.

Face blindness/prosopagnosia

I think Ben has difficulties recognising people. He gets faces muddled and thinks he recognises someone when in fact it is not the person at all. He shouts out loudly if he thinks someone looks like a character in a video he knows, at Heathrow airport recently he shouted "there's Dumbledoor" at a man with a long beard, I hope the man didn't know the Harry potter story at all!

Some people with autism have with face blindness (also called Prosopagnosia) they have a difficult time identifying people. Most people identify people by remembering other people's faces. People with face blindness don't seem to be able to do this, and thus must rely on other physical traits. One of the strengths of AS is attention to details.

In a recent interview Daniel Tannet describes how he finds it difficult to recognise someone he has only just met or someone he does not know well. Instead of regarding facial features as the way of recognising someone, Daniel like many others on the autistic spectrum notices other details:

"One hour after we leave today, and I will not remember what you look like. And I will find it difficult to recognize you, if I see you again. I will remember your handkerchief. And I will remember you have four buttons on your sleeve. And I'll remember the type of tie you're wearing. It's the details that I remember," Tammet tells Safer.

THE 'Q' FACTOR

http://60minutes.yahoo.com/segment/44/brain_man

I have great difficulty recognising faces and I recently did an online test for face blindness recently where I scored 32%. If you score les than 64% you are likely to have some degree of face blindness. I did the same test for recognition of cars and shoes where I scored 94% for shoes and 75% for cars. Taking the same test for cars and shoes reassured me that I do not have difficulty recognising shapes or with attention to detail, but I do have some problem recognising faces.

I recognise people using context, general body size/shape, hair, and the sound of their voice as my main clues. This is not as effective as the normal way of recognising people - by recognising a face. So sometimes I make mistakes. I might confuse a person for someone else, or fail to recognise and acknowledge someone I know. For example, recently I was talking to someone I know and it was only when I walked away that I thought they have put on weight. It was then that I realised I had confused them for someone else. Both men have a goatee beard and similar hair colour; I was using that as my means of identifying them. They were sitting down, so I could not use height as a factor and the environment was noisy so I could not rely so well on their voice. I was an embarrassing moment, I and I hope I did not say anything too obvious to show that I was talking to them thinking they were someone else!

I was out recently when I thought I recognised someone, I said hello and smiled and they said "I think not!" I must have been mistaken. They had a beard and glasses and I was using these factors to identify them as an acquaintance.

If someone changes their hair or appearance drastically, I find it very difficult to recognise them. Ladies who colour their hair frequently really confuse me. I also rely on types of car, hoping it will help me identify who people are. I think I see people I know, but I am often mistaken. I do not use names much when I speak to people, I hope by talking in general terms they won't notice that I might be confused as to who they are. If I am to introduce someone, I always start by naming the person I am with who I am confident about and just say "this is Malcolm" and stop. This generally prompts the other person to say who they are. This usually works. If it fails, I have a strategy which I use, I usually say that I have trouble with names and this gets me out of tricky situations. I'm really in trouble if I am having difficulty identifying the person I am with, they might have come over and started a conversation and I am inwardly panicking trying to identify them and how I know them! Then I say "who's going to start with the introductions?" and hope for the best! Having face blindness does make me even more nervous about social gatherings.

I find face blindness causes me difficulties keeping up with the plot in films and tv programmes. I am okay once I have identified a person by their voice, mannerisms, gait and by context, but it takes me extra effort to keep up. During programmes I frequently ask my husband to tell

THE 'Q' FACTOR

me who the people are. I also find it incredibly frustrating when someone you are watching something with asks "isn't that … from …." I think – how do I know?

In the face recognition of famous people test, I missed quite a few celebrities as you just see the face without much hair at all and they are not in context. I find I confuse 2 people who to me look similar. For example I find Matt Le Blanc similar to Matthew Broderick – although I am a huge Friends fan and when watching the tv show I have no difficulty recognising the characters. They all have very distinctive body shape, voices and mannerisms, so I particularly like Friends. Although the later series were harder as both Monica and Rachel had similar long straight hair, but their voices are very distinctive.

I find face blindness frustrating as I frequently think I have seen a character previously in a different episode, perhaps as a different character. This confuses and distracts me and I frequently have to rewind videos to refresh my memory of who is who!

While there is not much research on face blindness in people with autism, I think it might be more common than we realise.

Interpreting facial expression

As I am sure you probably know, this is something which people with autism find difficult. It is difficult enough to identify faces, but it is harder to interpret facial expression. I notice Ben tries to make sense of peoples expressions when he copies their faces and often contorts his face as he is doing it. He is very good at diffusing a situation when someone is angry, as he contorts his face to match theirs and it is actually really funny and usually brings a smile.

One of the most difficult things is understanding the difference between an extremely happy face and one which is very sad. Ben might actually laugh at someone who falls over and hurts themselves and cries. He finds this really funny. He gets facial expressions confused. We were on a train once and he saw a man who had a lot of lines on his forehead, I think they were frown lines. Ben asked why the man was crying – he was actually asleep!

Because of difficulty interpreting facial expression, it is difficult to understand how people are feeling and therefore the implied meaning of what they are saying. There are some people who seem to smile whatever they are talking about; this makes it difficult to understand their actual meaning. I once had a boss who smiled when she talked; it was very difficult to know if she was serious or joking about things.

THE 'Q' FACTOR

I find it difficult to understand teasing; someone says something serious with a smile. Do you believe the words or the smile? I find it difficult to tell if someone is being sarcastic. "You played the flute well last week" I might think they are teasing me or being sarcastic.

I learnt rules about eye contact when I was doing training for personnel. It is generally believed that if a person avoids eye contact then they are not confident or they could be not telling the truth. I find I prefer to watch someone's mouth rather than their eyes. I find eyes difficult as they flicker about and I find them distracting. I prefer to watch the mouth as this helps follow what the person is saying. I also find it very difficult if someone has eyes which do not both focus together. I usually find I am looking at the eye which is not focusing. I find it difficult to know which eye to look at, so looking at the mouth is easier. It is easier if someone wears glasses as the shadow or glare on the glasses takes the distraction away from the eyes. I have learnt to look at eyes as I know it is generally expected, but I also consciously look away from time to time as I have had people telling me that they think I am staring to intently. It is very difficult to get a balance.

When Ben was young, he did not make eye contact at all. His first speech therapist spent much time working on eye contact. In the first weeks during sessions, Ben got a reward if he made eye contact. He got to roll a ball down the ball run. This was his favourite toy at the therapy sessions. We borrowed the toy and used it at home in the same way. If we were trying to talk to Ben we used to say "Ben look at me" and when he did, he got to roll the ball. It was also important to say his name, so that he knew we were talking directly to him. I still use that approach as I notice Ben tunes out of conversations if he does not think it includes him. If you say, "everyone, put seat belts on", Ben won't do it. If you say, "Ben and everyone put seat belts on", then it works.

We don't have to ask Ben to look at us now, as he does engage with people really well. He prefers not to make eye contact, but he can do it. I wonder if he finds understanding the facial expressions distracting. It is easier to listen to the words and make sense of them, it takes the distracting face out of the process.

This is why people on the autistic spectrum prefer email contact to face to face. The written word is not confusing, you can read and then re read if you need to. You do not have to decipher the facial expression; email is detached and easier to process.

THE 'Q' FACTOR

Empathy

This leads me on to another difficulty which is empathy. Ben is actually more sad about the loss of the train rather than the people who are injured if he sees a train crash on the news.

One magic moment for me was when Ben saw and understood I was sad about our cat dying. I was a bit emotional and he came over and put is hand on my knee and asked me
"are you cold enough?" it was not the right language but the right emotional response.

I know if have difficulties with empathy. I force myself to try and empathise by remembering a situation I experienced and then transfer the feeling so that I can imagine how someone is feeling. I remember an incident when I was a child which I am still very ashamed of. A girl I was friendly with would not practise the recorder with me. I got so frustrated with her that I grabbed her thumb and bent it back until she screamed. I was surprised at her reaction and upset that I had hurt her. I did not mean to cause her extreme pain and was shocked at the result. I got in real trouble and was hauled into the Head Teachers room the next day and her Dad faced me and really told me off. I apologised but I can remember thinking it was a great amount of fuss. I could not imagine just how sore her thumb would have been. I was more upset about not playing the recorder than concerned about the pain of the other girl.

I have to force myself to try and consider other peoples feelings. I often speak and then think much later that I may have offended someone or I have been thoughtless. I spend a great amount of time apologising and trying to explain that I did not mean to offend.

I know my son is confused about empathy, he often has a smile on his face when someone else hurts themselves. I do not think this is because he is really happy at someone else's expense, but that he is confused about what emotion to show and how to understand what the other person is feeling.
I know I look to others to see their responses and copy their expressions, I think my son does that too. I have written more about emotional responses in a later section.

Medical appointments

Medical appointments can be very traumatic for any family. We have had a few bad experiences in hospitals with Ben.

Blood Test at local hospital

The first hospital visit was to our local hospital for a routine blood test as an outpatient. (Hillingdon Hospital). Ben was sent a notice of the time to attend the ward for the blood test.

On arrival at the hospital I tried to identify the nurse who would be conducting the test. I wanted to speak to her about how to handle Ben. I was anxious to avoid Ben having a crisis and getting upset. If he got stressed his behaviour would deteriorate and he would harm himself by repeatedly banging his head on the ground or hitting himself and making a very high pitched screech. This behaviour was no good for either him or other children in the ward.

The nurse on duty did not take any time to listen to my requests. We were kept waiting for 4 hours in total, this is unacceptable for any child – but totally impossible for an Autistic child.

After 1 ½ hours Ben had "magic cream" put on the back of his hands. He was very sensitive to anything on his hands and found this very distressing. The explanation by the nurse would have meant nothing to him. She explained in detail what was going to happen. This made Ben more stressed. I asked her to just carry out the procedure and I would deal with Ben. She insisted on explaining that the magic cream would not hurt and it would help him have his tiny prick on his hand. He was told he would get a sticker afterwards! All the language and time taken to explain caused more harm than good. Ben became more and more upset.

Waiting with children in the hot and crowded play area was very hard. Other parents glared at me as I sat with a child who was quite and wild and angry. I could do very little with him. I was tempted to take him home and abandon the experience, but I knew that I would not get Ben back into the building.

Finally we were called for the blood test. Again the soft approach was used and long explanations given to Ben. I had him in a vice lock and hung onto him to keep him still. The Nurse eventually listened to me, but I had to demand that she took the blood and let us go. Ben screamed and drew quite a crowd at the window of the room.

The experience was a very stressful one. A routine blood test caused great distress and trauma. Ben had a bad week following the visit. He was unsettled by the events and it was difficult to bring routine and normality back into his world.

THE 'Q' FACTOR

Children with autism do not have a concept of time or of turn taking. Ben was told to wait and play until it was his turn. In his world he would have been scared and felt out of place. He was in unfamiliar surroundings and with strangers.

Routine and familiarity is very important to children – especially those with Autism. If a child is to have hospital visits, it would be of benefit to visit the ward without any medical investigation or treatment taking place. This would allow the child to familiarise themselves with the environment and have a positive and unthreatening experience in the hospital. If a negative or bad experience is had, then the parent would struggle to get the child back into the building as children with Autism may have very acute memories for detail and places.

Children with autism may also have very sensitive hearing and be distressed by noisy wards. Care should be taken using loud equipment – noisy hand dryers may cause real distress if set off while a child is in the cloakroom.

It would be of benefit if hospital workers were aware of the severe distress behaviours, which may be exhibited by a child with Autism. Head banging on the floor or with their hand, hitting himself or herself or the wall, pacing, swaying, loud humming or screaming or screeching. Any children with Autistic Spectrum disorders may demonstrate some or all of these. The behaviour is distressing for the child, family members or the staff, but it does affect other children and patients. Having a quiet room for such children would be of great benefit. A quiet "time out zone" allows calming and reassuring time for the child and prevents the stress building up to such an extent that the bizarre behaviours be demonstrated.

If the staff had more understanding of Autism, they could also reassure the other children and families and help prevent some of the judgement and criticism from other people.

Children can become frightened of a fiery child, and hospital visits do unfortunately often bring out the worst traits of Autism, as there is so much anxiety.

The long visit to Hillingdon Hospital was made very difficult not only by Ben and his difficulties, but the judgement and criticism of other people.

Brain Scan at Central Middlesex Hospital

As part of the routine investigations Ben was booked in for a brain scan.

My sister came with me for moral support, as I was very worried about how Ben would cope and worried that I would be too emotional to deal with his needs. Children with Autism or any communication disorder are in tune to parent's emotions without the need for language. My stress or anxiety would cause Ben's behaviour to deteriorate

On arrival at the hospital I spoke to the nurse about Ben's needs. We were shown to a waiting area, fortunately there were only 2 other children waiting before us.

Despite my request to keep language simple and the information given to Ben to a minimum, the nurse came at him with a loaded syringe of sedative and a tirade of language. Ben ran away, the nurse cornered him and after more explanations she tried to administer the dose. The result was that Ben was covered by the sticky liquid. This further distressed him as common to autism is a dislike of touching unusual substances and a dislike of mess.

The nurse suggested putting the sedative in a drink. We put the medicine in a half empty can of coke to entice Ben.

It took 1 hour to encourage him to drink the liquid. We had been advised that the sedative would cause Ben to be drowsy and collapse in sleep.

The medication caused the opposite in Ben (we later found this to be the case with many other drugs suggested to cause sleep or sedation – again common to children with an autistic spectrum disorder).

Ben proceeded to lunge around the room as if he was drunk. He laughed and fell over a few times, but no sign of sleep!

Eventually after many hours the nurse suggested an alternative sedation as again I requested that he be sedated because we would not be able to bring him back to the hospital, as he would refuse to enter the building.

We were taken to the ward and a suppository was prepared. Again the nurse came to explain the procedure to Ben, I begged her to "just do it."

Ben fell asleep after falling head first off the end of the bed!

It was 4 pm and when we advised the nurse that he was finally asleep, she said "oh, the Doctor goes off duty at 4, so you may have to come back another day!"

I carried Ben along many corridors to the room for the brain scan, while walking along noisy corridors, he woke up! The Doctor kindly agreed to carry out the brain scan. He stuck electrodes on Ben in a "hell raiser head" fashion. If Ben had been awake the entire wire assortment would have been ripped off in one movement. The brain scan was done just as Ben woke up and pulled off the wires.

THE 'Q' FACTOR

We were advised that the result may not be conclusive, as the medication finally used to sedate Ben was so strong that it would affect the readings! This was frustrating news to us and Ben was a very unhappy boy after the experience.

It took 6 weeks to get the glue out of his hair following sticking the electrodes on his head.

On arrival at the hospital I tried to explain to the nurse that Ben needed simple language and limited explanations about medical procedure. This advice was ignored.

Parents know their children and much time can be saved if their wishes are adhered to.

If a child has had an adverse reaction to medication or sedation then it could be that other medications may cause bizarre reactions or behaviour. We were already aware that Phernagan a product that can be used to induce sleep caused the reverse in Ben. This information may have prevented us spending so much time waiting for a drug to sedate Ben, a stronger drug could have been prescribed for him from the outset.

As children with Autism may have such bizarre and differing behaviour to normal children, more time than average should be allowed for such investigations and tests.

Operation at Great Ormond Street Hospital

At the age of 6 Ben had to undergo surgery to correct a congenital soft mucal palette. The condition caused him to speak with a very nasal tone and food would get stuck at the back of his throat. Concerned about the nasal quality of Ben's speech, the school speech therapist referred Ben to the specialist clinic at Great Ormond Street Hospital for their assessment.

Following 2 out patient visits to the hospital to attend the Cleft palette clinic and see the plastic surgeon the operation was booked. The initial visits to the hospital had been fairly pleasant for Ben as he enjoyed the journey by underground train. Ben's school speech therapist accompanied us and this greatly helped when meeting the professionals. The tests needed to assess Ben's extent of palette condition had already been done in part by the speech therapist and she could advise the specialists in the jargon and technical terms needed.

I used the lessons learned in our previous hospital visits to try and make the visit as bearable for Ben as possible. I had a reward for him – his favourite of the 7 dwarfs to cuddle as he waited for the appointment; we went on a long and roundabout journey taking as many trains as we could to get to the hospital. This made the event more fun for Ben.

THE 'Q' FACTOR

The operation was booked in November 98. I was 8 months pregnant with my third child. We arrived at the hospital, Ben was in good spirits. The efforts made to make the out patient appointments fun, made our "sleep visit" to hospital less of a trauma for Ben. The first day was spent with admission procedure.

Ben enjoyed playing in the play room. We had little sleep, as we were in a ward with 3 other children without their parents. They were distressed and needed reassurance. My advice would be to allow and encourage parents to stay with any young children! I spent much time reassuring and comforting other people's children.

On the morning of the operation I asked when Ben would be taken to theatre. He was number 6 on the list! I had advised the Surgeon that he could not wait so long without food and waiting for something he did not understand would be difficult. He was due to be taken at 2pm. He wanted to eat and did not want the "magic cream" on his hand for the entire morning. The nursing staff also insisted that he wore a gown for most of the time. He was not at all comfortable about being in a gown. Children with Autism may not even like to remove a sweater if they began the day wearing it. Changing clothing is something they may not like.

Ben coped fairly well, but was getting more and more anxious as the time went by. The pre med was administered at 12pm. The medication made him hallucinate. Instead of relaxing him, he tried to leap off the bed and later the trolley. He tore at the needle in his had for medication. He was wheeled to theatre and had to be physically held onto the trolley as he lunged off the end. He struggled until he was put to sleep. But after the operation Ben awoke in the same state.

Such a reaction to a pre med is not uncommon in children with an autistic spectrum disorder. Adverse reaction although not an allergic reaction to certain drugs seems to be common and should be considered when preparing for medical procedures.

It was 5pm when we were wheeled back to the ward. Following Ben's behaviour in recovery a room had been prepared for us at the end of the ward to minimise disruption to other children.

I had to lie on the bed with Ben holding his hands away from his mouth as he tore at his stitches and could have pulled them all out. He was very upset. I begged the nursing staff to help him.

After an exhausting hour of trauma medication was administered by suppository. The usual saga of the nurse explaining in full began and I almost screamed, "just do it! I will deal with him".

Ben finally went into a fitful sleep.

THE 'Q' FACTOR

The first night and most of the next day were spent dealing with a disturbed child. The anaesthetic caused Ben to be sick many times. He was not a cooperative patient. The tiny bowl provided to catch the vomit was useless as he lunged around the bed, off the bed and around the room in distress as he vomited. I was assisted the first time I had to change his bedding, but on further occasions I was left to cope.

Despite being 8 months pregnant and having a very difficult child I was given no respite or assistance. At 7am the following morning my husband arrived and I at least got a shower and managed to make myself some breakfast. That was the first I had eaten since the previous morning!

It seemed as if the staff were afraid of us and did not come near the room.

Ben refused his painkiller as it was not the calpol he was used to. I disguised the medication in a drink. This was not technically allowed by the hospital, but one nurse bent the rules as after 2 ½ days, she had begun to understand Ben.

The first 3 days were very difficult and we had little support from staff. The hospital routine and procedure were designed around a child who could understand and cooperate with staff and parents. Other parents could leave their child asleep and go to the parents restaurant for a meal or to the shop. I could not leave Ben unsupervised for very long. At times the run to the other end of the ward for clean bedding was a worry as Ben could have fallen out of bed or even run away.

A child with an autistic spectrum disorder needs 24-hour care and supervision to prevent them harming themselves or others. Some respite or help for parents should be available in hospitals.

Our 7 day stay in Great Ormond Street was very difficult, but the operation was a total success and has benefited Ben to such an extent that his speech sounds normal and his eating is much more normal too. It was certainly worth putting him through the procedure.

I can look back and reflect on the experiences related – at the time, each one caused real distress. Parents of children with additional support needs or disabilities, especially those with Autism feel vulnerable and isolated. We look to professionals for support and advice. People are quick to judge parents of children with Autism as the disability is hidden. The child just looks out of control or badly behaved.   Insensitive comments can do incredible damage to the whole family including siblings and parents.

<u>Tips for dealing with children with autism at medical appointments</u>

THE 'Q' FACTOR

Some degree of flexibility in procedure and routine should be allowed for a child with autism. (Such as allowing medication in to be given in a drink, allowing the favourite toy in pre theatre or recovery)

Pre hospital visits for familiarisation with the surroundings and staff are a good idea. These could be done in advance of any medical appointment and then routinely to keep the child familiar with the hospital setting.

As familiarity is especially important to autistic children, parents could be encouraged to bring in familiar items from home, such as posters, books, toys, favourite video or cassette. It would also be of benefit to suggest a supply of the child's normal pain relief and some of his favourite food, drinks and snacks.

On a practical note, more pyjamas and changes of clothes than normal for both Mum and child should be brought in.

Any waiting time should be kept to a minimum. If possible allow autistic children to wait and stay in quiet surroundings with toys such as trains, cars, bricks and drawing materials.

I wish medical staff would listen to parent's specific requests and medical history. Any previous experiences of reactions to medication should be noted as they might be relevant to the current visit.

If the child needs to use sign language, basic signs could be used by hospital staff.

All staff should be aware that if they wear any kind of uniform, this may be associated by the child as someone who administers pain. A child with autism might not distinguish between a surgeon, physiotherapist or cleaner if they all wear uniform. A member of staff may get a better response from the child if they were to temporarily remove the white coat or overall. Children with autism use visual clues to make sense of their world and surroundings. Picture sequence cards could be used for the child to follow instructions.

Keeping the surroundings quiet and avoiding slang or generalisations, could help a child with autism understand the situation better. It is important to speak to the child on his level, and not to stand up tall and speak down to them.

It would help to allow child to finish activities before removing them for the appointment or testing eg. "Put your train into the station and then we can look at your eyes can't we?"

Or

"Put one more brick on your tower then we can go in here".

THE 'Q' FACTOR

A befriending person or a counsellor would be of great assistance to families in hospitals. Parents of autistic children feel very isolated and may choose to stay alone rather than try to mix with other patient's and families. The effort of explaining the child's bizarre behaviour to others with no understanding of the condition is often difficult and overwhelming. Respite for parents would be of great benefit.

Keeping changes of personnel to a minimum would help greatly, as children with autism need the familiarity.

Charities such as Crossroads may be able to assist with families in hospitals

After our trip to great Ormond street hospital, Ben was phobic of anyone wearing a white coat. I could not walk him past the butchers, hair dressers or near any one wearing painter overalls without a major stress reaction. He would pull away, scream, try to run off and really panic in case he was to get an injection or treatment like he did in hospital.

We have had our fair share of hospital appointments. Even getting a routine blood test becomes a major trauma. Waiting times, busy waiting rooms, sensory overload, change in routine, having to remove items of clothing, the insistent medic who ignoring the mothers requests, MUST tell the patient absolutely every thing which is going to happen to them, in lovely long words and jargon, standing with a syringe it is all very traumatic.

These traumatic moments only cause more difficulties, as it makes future appointments very difficult to manage. We had used bribery, star charts, social stories, stickers, rewards, train rides, and more to overcome some of Ben's fears. After the hospital visit to great Ormond street and then one recently at a local hospital for tooth extraction, I have done a few dummy trips to hospital, just to go in, do something nice like buy a chocolate bar from the wonderful shop and then leave again.

Dentists

My son does not like going to the dentist. We have had difficulty getting him to clean his teeth and then we had severe problems getting him to visit a dentist. With much patience and wonderful understanding staff, over time we have made progress in this area with Ben.

Having a toothbrush in your mouth is causes difficulty if you have sensory issues. Ben has some touch sensitivities, and I think he has difficulty tolerating some tastes. I had to find toothpaste he could tolerate and a toothbrush which was soft enough for him to cope with. When he was very young, I used to distract him with his favourite toy and then try and clean his

THE 'Q' FACTOR

teeth at the same time. I was not always successful as he soon learnt what I was about to do and he has an amazing strength in his jaw. I could not force him to let me clean his teeth or allow me to even put a brush in his mouth or this might have caused him more distress and then he would struggle ever using a toothbrush. As usual we motivated him using his favourite activities. The whole procedure from starting to accustomise Ben with the tools for the job to actually being able to successfully brush his teeth took months.

I found a Thomas the tank engine toothbrush and tooth paste which made things easier. I bought a whole lot of the brushes so I had plenty of spares. I figured we would end up throwing a few away. I gave Ben one brush to hold and fiddle with while I tried to clean the teeth. It took a few days of letting him play with a toothbrush before he would let me use one in his mouth. Rather than let him have a toothbrush the whole time, I did put it away after each attempt to clean his teeth, so that it was always interesting. The brush Ben held was rammed inside many objects; he loved posting it in the strangest places. He pushed it through his brio train tunnel with great delight, especially if the cat tried to grab the other end. One was binned after he put it in his potty as he used it, and one was lost down the side of the sofa. Ben would have put one in the video player if we didn't already have a video guard – this was purchased after Ben put his weetabix inside the video player! Incidentally, when I saw Ben taking the video guard off the player and inserting a different Thomas video when one had finished, I soon stopped using it, gladly the weetabix phase had passed!

I put the toothpaste on his favourite biscuit, so he could get used to the taste. At first, he screamed at me for ruining his favourite biscuit, but luckily he did like the taste of the toothpaste. I remember checking with the health visitor as Ben went through a stage where he would try and grab the tube and suck as much of it out as possible before I managed to get it off him. I was assured that this would not do him any permanent fluoride overload if we stopped the activity as soon as we could.

We started cleaning teeth in front of a Thomas video; I ignored the advice from the health visitor with this as she said we should only clean his teeth in the bathroom. I found if I tried that, then Ben would object to going in the bathroom for anything else. He associated it with the trauma of having his teeth brushed. Obviously we couldn't have the situation where he would not go into the bathroom at all, so I decided to relax that rule and try to clean teeth in a place where Ben himself was calm and relaxed; I thought that would be the best time to try and get him used to the toothbrush.

I actually remember carrying a toothbrush out with us, and getting Ben to use it when I could. This worked quite well one particular day, and I think we did actually do some effective teeth cleaning. We were going for a ride on trains. I used to spend one afternoon a week with Ben riding on the tube trains. We used to buy a ticket for 1 zone and then he and I would get on any train, the first one which arrived in the station and we would ride backwards and forwards 2 stops each way and do this for as long as I could stand it. This was Ben's absolute favourite activity. I think that the true train spotter does not have to have a destination in mind; just the delight of riding on a train while admiring other passing trains and track brings the enjoyment!

I think sheer determination combined with a relaxed and alternative approach to teeth cleaning meant that we did manage to conquer the fear of the tooth brush. We progressed onto sticker charts; board maker checklists, visual time tables showing morning and evening routines and now years on, Ben has an electric toothbrush which he uses independently every day without prompting. It is part of his routine and he does it really well. When you are going through the early stages building up to the large task, it seems that you make little progress very quickly and it is difficult to persevere, but gradually one step at a time, breaking things down into manageable stages means you can conquer even the most challenging and daunting activities or tasks.

I can apply this to myself and to my children. I use the same step by step approach with dog training too and it seems to work. You see the required behaviour and work out a way of breaking it down into small stages. Gradually you build up a pattern of behaviour you want.

It is usually easier to apply this approach to other people but I find it more difficult to use it myself if there is something I find particularly overwhelming. I have to confess that I am dentist phobic. I have actually got worse over time. The uniform the staff wear, the smell of the chemical products, the lighting and equipment and the sound of other people receiving treatment are all difficult to cope with if you have sensory issues. I have sat in dentist waiting rooms literally shaking with fear and have actually made many excuses not to go. I do not go to the dentist for regular check ups; I only go if I feel pain. I know this is not the best way to have healthy teeth, but I do not like the trauma of the experience.

I have had some particularly traumatic visits to the dentist both as a child and also as an adult. I am so bad now, that I cannot watch a programme on television if they show any dentist work. Even the animated film "finding Nemo" has scenes which I cannot watch or listen to. If people speak about experiences of going to the dentist, I put my hand over my ears.

When we were young my Mum took us to the dentist each school holiday. At first I did not mind going at all, but when I experienced my first filling, I really hated going. The dentist did not use pain relief at all. I have one upper tooth which was shaped in such a way that it ground into a lower tooth, this caused problems and I ended up having the lower tooth filled repeatedly. It felt to me as if the dentist was slowing making patterns on my tooth and it hurt so much. He used to say, just raise your arm if it hurts and I will stop. I knew this was not true as I would raise my arm as soon as he put the metal drill into my mouth and started work, I find the vibration of the drill and the noise extremely painful.

I have had to stop writing this as I am feeling very unwell at the thought.

Once I found a dentist who used pain relief, I found it easier to cope with the visits, but it is sheer determination which gets me through it. I went intermittently only when I really had to due to severe tooth ache. However, since my last visit I have not been back in 5 years. I cannot bring myself to write about it.

I have to mention here that the there are some good dentist and medical experiences too. We have a local special care dentistry service which is wonderful. What a difference it makes when a child with autism is understood and things are booked accordingly.

In advance of the visit, the dentist asked us what the best time of day would be for an appointment.

We completed a form and answered questions about likes and dislikes, things that Ben finds difficult and special instructions around how to make the visit easier. At Ben's first visit, the dentist asked my son if he wanted him to wear the mask and he did not wear the uniform jacket. Ben got to take along his favourite soft toys and they were included as part of the process. The first visit was purely to familiarise us with the surgery, the staff, the equipment, the dreaded chair etc. No pain was inflicted at all! Ben came away saying,

"Can I come here every Friday?" high praise indeed.
This was short hand for "can I come here and miss maths every Friday and play with stuff please?"

I might actually ask if I can attend the dentist clinic myself – or maybe not!

THE 'Q' FACTOR

Peer pressure

This is something families of an autistic child actually long for!
I longed for the day when Ben would come home with his shirt hanging out and that teenage slouch. For muddy knees and that well known rolling of the eyes – I longed to hear the phrase "everyone else has one"

We do now have the shirt hanging out, which is wonderful, as it used to be neatly tucked in every morning and would not be worn showing under the school jumper. Now the t shirts are often longer than the jumper and they are left hanging loose over the trousers.

Ben now has a mobile phone like all this friends. He has told us that the other kids in his school taxi have a mobile, but he did not really want one just to be the same as the others. As he now likes to go into town and spend his pocket money, and we are trying to build his independence, I might be very useful that he has a mobile phone. What is amusing however is that he turns it off after every use, he only uses it to phone his brother and granny – which he does loudly pacing up and down while we are watching a video with Lauren or doing her homework! Then the phone is turned off, put in the box and put away in his bedroom.

At 15 Ben has never had a sleep over
Never used a swear word

Never been bowling or to the cinema with a pal –
without a paid minder!
Never smoked a cigarette
Never been on the bus on his own
Only has visitors who are paid to look after him!

In Orkney Ben does have some independence,
Dial a Bus is great as he can go to town and
spend his pocket money – this is thanks to much
work done by Ben's Personal Assistant through
direct payments. He can now go into a shop,
spend his money, even ask for something if he
can't see it. I went into the local charity shop
(Ben's favourite shop) with him once. It seems he
is very well known in there and the staff told me he
is "the most polite boy they have had" a great
compliment.

So although we have things which make us sad,
we have a lot to be thankful for. Gladly peer
pressure worries that some parents have do not
worry us. We do worry that he might not have
many friends, but he probably won't make friends
with the "wrong crowd." Ben will never be a bully,
he will never knowingly harm another child, and he
will never tease someone mercilessly or be rude
to a teacher or police man. He has respect for
adults, and although he gets things wrong, he isn't
knowingly malicious or belligerent.

The best social time for Ben was when he
attended our local school for 1 year. This was the
first time he had been at a local school as

previously he attended a school 22 miles away from home and got taken by taxi every day. When going to Firth, Ben got to walk to school for the first time. Around that time we also invested in a "rebound Therapy equipment" a large trampoline. It is the best thing we have bought our kids and I think most families who have a child on the autistic spectrum have got a trampoline! It was a babe magnet in the village. Kids could see it as we live up a hill and so for one whole summer, every day after school we had a stream of kids knocking at the door "is Ben home?" We knew they just wanted to go on the trampoline, but it was the best time for Ben has he had friends pop round. Now there are 6 other trampolines in the village! But since he moved to secondary school we don't have pals pop round.

Inappropriate behaviour

You hear this term usually when professionals are around. The term Inappropriate behaviour covers a huge range. It can take many forms, it could be talking too loudly, fidgeting, pacing, rocking to full blown tantrums in the middle of the supermarket.

The inappropriate behaviour can also be invading someone's space or getting things wrong socially. Ben wants to be friends, but doesn't always know how to join in a conversation or get someone's attention. When he was small he used to pull a girls hair, now he just stands too close to someone or copies them when hey are talking just because he wants to join in.

The most embarrassing form of this inappropriate behaviour is of course the major meltdown. Ben can make the most ear piercing scream, and put so much energy to throwing his whole body to the floor and kicking and screaming and act like the worst unhappy toddler you have ever met. This is fine when it happens at home, but it can erupt anytime. We have learnt to mange the frustrations Ben has and see the signs when he is about to erupt. I can usually diffuse the situation by talking about his favourite subject DMUs or when he was smaller I used to start singing his favourite song. The major meltdown can happen when the stress and anxiety levels are too high. The trigger for the actual moment of crisis might be something fairly trivial. It is almost as if there is a pressure gauge in side and it reaches the point of maximum pressure and then the top has to blow.

Inappropriate behaviour can also be just wearing the wrong clothes at the wrong time or carrying a favourite item about. At the age of 8 Ben's older brother asked if Ben could not meet him from school. He was embarrassed as at that time Ben carried a Barbie doll everywhere. He loves to flick the hair. Now he has jelly cat mermaids. He flicks them. Its quite therapeutic, I tried it myself.

Ben likes Lazy Town and Fifi and the flower tots. These programmes are designed to be enjoyed by pre school children. Ben loves to watch them and he carries characters from the programmes in his back pack. At 15 he now realises it is not appropriate that he carries these things about. When he is stressed however, he carries them anyway, and doesn't seem to worry about what other people might think, he just finds them comforting.

I am conscious all the time about my behaviour and actions. I worry that I am conforming to expectations and that I am getting things right. I try to avoid group situations or large gatherings unless I am very comfortable with the people there. I have to force myself to attend something new as I find it very difficult defining how I should behave. If I am on a group or a committee, and there is a change of personnel I find it very difficult and I worry about how I come across until I know the person and I can see how the change affects the group dynamic.

I spend time observing people around me and copy how they behave. I find I identify a strong character who I usually admire and then I mimic their behaviour. I can take on characteristics and find I can sound quite like them. I am so worried about behaving inappropriately; it is quite time consuming and absorbing.

I am worried that I stand too close to people and one thing I have noticed about myself is that I have the tendency to interrupt when people are speaking. I am consciously trying to correct this as I can guess that it is very annoying.

I think I possibly talk at people at length when I am speaking about something I feel passionately about. I am aware that I have this tendency and again I monitor it all the time. I am probably potentially at my most boring when I am speaking about access issues. While I was on the training course at Heriot Watt University to learn to become an Access Auditor, I was aware that some people rattled on about something they felt strongly about and they tended to bore people and leave the rest of the group behind; expressions glazed over. I try to be aware of this and keep my contributions short and try to avoid anecdotes too much.

On the course, it was amusing to watch the screen at the front of the room while the palentypist

THE 'Q' FACTOR

scribed the entire lecture. When one person spoke, they typed the persons name and as track record had showed that they spoke at length usually about something we had heard before, the words "blah, blah, blah" came up on the screen! I would be mortified if those words were typed alongside my name in a meeting!

Inappropriate behaviour can be simply boring people around you too much about your favourite subject or it could be one of the ritualistic behaviours used by some people on the autistic spectrum.

Self stimulating behaviour

Behaviours exhibited by some people on the autistic spectrum might be directly related to the sensory difficulties the person is experiencing or being exposed to. Some people have difficulty with sensory overload which is too many different sensory experiences at any one time.
There might also be difficulty in processing particular sensory information. Self stimulating behaviour may be done by people on the autistic spectrum as a way of reminding themselves of their body extremities. For example, bumping into objects or standing too close to people, flapping, flicking and hitting parts of the body might be used by some people who have difficulty with body awareness. Rocking might be used by someone who experiences difficulty with balance or awareness of how their body fits into their environment.
Self stimulating behaviour is also used as a way of coping, as a sort o stress relief in an overpowering world which bombards the senses. Rocking is a soothing movement and it can help tune out unwanted sensory overload. Many families affected by autism have trampolines. These are a great stress reliever and a good way to express frustrations while helping balance and coordination. Buying a garden or indoor swing is also a good way of allowing a behaviour which brings relief to someone, but it is more socially acceptable than someone rocking in a corner.

THE 'Q' FACTOR

Ben flaps, paces, claps, rocks, hums and does a number of ritualistic behaviours which are totally fine with us at home but not always acceptable when out. I have tried them all, and when he gets too involved in them, I mimic them back to him which he finds really amusing. You have to watch other children mimicking though as he finds that very upsetting. I have learnt that it is best not to restrict him using these behaviours, but best to channel them.

The pacing we use as dog training. He walks the dog up and down. The dog gets some individual attention and exercise and Ben gets to do his pacing behaviour.

Some toys are particularly good for flapping or flicking. Ben has always liked rag dolls with long hair. We have some rag doll Jellycat mermaids which Ben loves. He has collected them all and enjoys playing with them as toys and also gets genuine stress relief from flicking and flapping them. It is unusual for a 15 year old boy to carry mermaid toys about, so we allow the mermaids at home, in the car and comfortable places like church, but Ben usually puts them in his back pack when out. But it is reassuring for him to know that they are there.

I have also found that using one of Ben's favourite toys is a good way of communicating with him. If he doesn't want to go out on a family outing, we invite the mermaids to go and talk through them.

They tell Ben that they would really like to go along and sit with their best friends in the car. I also use the mermaids to find out how Ben is feeling. He will tell Molly mermaid what happened at school and may find it easer to use the mermaid to describe his emotions.

I find that I wring my hands. I have even developed eczema in my palms where I force my hands together and rub them so much. If I were to try and describe why I do this, I think it helps me concentrate; it is an automatic behaviour which feels pleasant. It keeps the circulation going in my hands and tunes out the pins and needles I get when I get too much sensory information to process at once or when I get tired.

I also scratch the sides of my thumbs with my finger nails. I do this more when I am anxious. I usually do it when I am worried and I will scratch until it bleeds. It is only when I can see the blood that I feel any sensation. It is almost as if the visual sign gives me the clue to experience a feeling.

I can do both my self stimulation behaviours while I am with other people. They do not usually notice as I keep my hands under the desk or in my pockets. My parents used to notice my thumbs were bleeding and sore, I would get told off about that. I do try very hard to stop it and I can manage it better as I have got older.

THE 'Q' FACTOR

When I feel the need to wring my hands or scratch my thumbs, I try to substitute this behaviour with tapping my big toe inside my shoe. I learnt to do this when at school. At orchestra practise, my music teacher told us to stop tapping our feet to keep the rhythm right. He said that if everyone tapped their feet in time to the music then all that could be heard would be tapping and it would be very distracting to see feet tapping at different times. He told us to tap our toes inside our shoes as no one could see this. I took his advice and use that technique as a stress reliever. I concentrate on my toe, think about the rhythm and tune out the stress of the situation. When I am consciously tapping my toe inside my shoe, I do feel it calms me down and helps with anxiety.

Hyper sensitivity

People on the autistic spectrum may have different sensitivities to others. Any of the senses can be affected, just one or all.

Temple Grandin in her book "thinking in pictures" describes how she is very sensitive to clothing. She has to wash clothes repeatedly before wearing them and sometimes wears things inside out as the seams feel like broken glass on her skin. My son hates wearing jeans or clothes which feel restrictive. He sticks to jogging trousers and tee shirts. I don't think he would like wearing a tie at all. It means he doesn't follow fashion but he is comfortable. I think he has so much to cope with to get through each day that I don't insist on him wearing certain clothes. It only becomes an issue for a formal occasion such as a wedding, but gladly we have got by with one pair of elasticised jeans which he will now tolerate for a short period of time.

Incidentally, if I buy Ben new clothes, I wash them first and sometimes I just put in them in his cupboard in among the familiar things so they start to smell right. If we find a coat or item which he really likes, I sometimes buy the next size too so that when he grows out of his favourite item of clothing, I can wash the new one and he usually won't notice the difference.

THE 'Q' FACTOR

At nearly 16 years old, my son tip toe walks, this may be the result of hypersensitivity. When he was small he did not like walking on sand or on wet surfaces. He developed tip toe walking so he did not have to stand fully on an undesirable surface. There is no physical reason why he tip toe walks, he has been examined by a physiotherapist, but it seems to be a choice he makes. It has become a habit but it probably started as young as 2 years old. I remember he did not walk until we went on holiday to cornwall. He crawled everywhere or relied on me to carry him. The feeling of the sand must have been unpleasant on his hands, so he stood up and walked – on tip toes! He has done this ever since. We also had to teach him to walk in puddles! Most parents spend time telling their children not to walk in puddles, we actively spent hours encouraging Ben to jump in puddles just for fun. We also had to make him try to walk through leaves when they fell off the trees in autumn. He will do this now, but very reluctantly and he makes facial expressions which confirm that he does not like the sensation of scrunching on leaves or anything underfoot.

Ben and I are affected by sounds. Ben has hypersensitive hearing. He cannot tolerate some high pitch sounds. It physically hurts his ears. Alarms are the worst for him. Malcolm had to change the ring tone on his mobile phone because if it rang, Ben would run screaming until it was stopped. I do not like the feed back you get from microphones; it hurts my ears so I can understand how Ben feels. Malcolm is learning the bodhran, he is really good at it. Ben cannot cope with the sound if it is in a small room. I was in the bedroom and Malc was practising, Ben ran screaming upstairs because he couldn't past the sound and find me in the bedroom. He wanted to tell me something, but couldn't cope with the noise, so he went away upset.

Hypersensitivity is real. It is a painful experience and should not be dismissed. Many parents and teachers try to ignore it and make a child suffer greatly in the process. Putting a child with hypersensitive hearing next to the computer equipment in the classroom would not be a good idea, tuning out the noise is difficult enough, but the constant humming would hurt your ears after a while, kind of like constant tinnitus.

I went to a local seminar and the only seats left were in the front row right behind the projector and lap top. I asked if I could sit at the back, but the organiser wanted to sit there so she asked me to sit at the front. I tried it, I sat in the front row for a couple of moments, but I had to move. I knew my time would be completely wasted if I sat there, as all I could hear was the humming of the projector and I also have difficulty sitting in the front row of a meeting room as I don't like the feeling of peoples eyes behind me, also I look at other people all the time for visual clues for what they are doing, are they standing up, are they laughing, looking at the presenters face, at the over head screen, at each other, out of the window at a sign on the wall, are they packing things away, taking notes, or whatever. So I had to cope with 2 very difficult things and this is something to consider when thinking about children on the autistic spectrum. It might be that a teacher likes to sit a child who might fidget or be a bit disruptive in the front row, this might cause the child real discomfort.

Sometimes when my son reacts adversely to a situation, it might be because he finds something about it painful. Going to clubs such as Boys Brigade means wearing a sweater and cap. The sweater had a very tight neck so that was one reason why he didn't like going. It can be difficult to find the reason why, but it is worth considering that when a child might be behaving in an inappropriate way, they might find something painful or uncomfortable.

Ben used to love going in the minibus to school. He had a driver who made it fun and went off quite happily. We had a change of driver and Ben decided he didn't want to go to school. He would gesture at the mini bus when it arrived and when it left. The driver actually reported an incident saying Ben threw a stone at the minibus. When we unravelled the situation. I spoke to Ben, and looked at where he was sitting in the bus, it turned out that the window next to him had a slight crack where the wind was whistling in. That explained it, that would annoy Ben and could have been physically painful if the wind was rushing down his ear. The driver taped the gap and the problem was solved. It was no longer a problem.

There could be a number of reasons why a child on the autistic spectrum behaves in an inappropriate way, I have heard of a child who acted inappropriately in class and the teacher contacted the National Autistic Society Helpline. They helped investigate the difficulty and it turned out that at 1.45 every day, the heating clicked on and the radiators crackled. This sound might have been painful to the child and they could not explain but it made them feel uncomfortable and so their behaviour changed. The problem could be solved by clicking the heating on when the children are out in the playground or giving the child a set of headphones or something to listen to at that time every day, so they didn't hear the sound. That could be the time to practice class singing or brain gym.

Hypersensitivity to touch could cause a number of difficulties, there are times in school when you have to touch things which would be very uncomfortable. My son used to hate play dough, he would not touch sand and hated physical contact. Again, by using his interests and passions, at school and at home, we worked on conditioning and he learnt to tolerate these things.

I do not like the sensation of cold meat or baking on my hands. In cooking I hated making pastry as you have to tolerate the margarine and flour in your fingernails. One week we had a different teacher, who taught me to use a knife to mix the dough. That was wonderful, I still use a knife when I make pastry now and I love having a dish washer because all those difficult dishes I can put straight in the dish washer and I don't have to touch the dough or meat products! My daughter always loved getting her hands in the baking bowls, I don't understand it, but I am grateful to her because she has fun doing the jobs I hate.

I do not like light touch. If my husband puts sun cream on my back, he has to remember to be firm with his touch or it literally feels like an insect on my back it is a very unpleasant sensation.

Because of my own sensitivities, it helps me understand my son. I use firm touch with him and make it clear when I am going to put my arm around him to hug him. He does not like a hug to creep up unexpectedly. If my son hurts himself, he hits himself in the place it hurts, this sounds dreadful, but if he hates light touch like I do, then he might find it reassuring to feel the hard sensation and it might help him cope with the pain.

I used a tens machine when I was in labour and the midwife told me not to turn it right up as that would be too painful, but I did. I hated the light sensation it gave if it was on too low, but once it was pulsing hard into my back on the maximum setting, it was reassuring, I could feel it and I liked the rhythm it gave and I tuned into that to cope with the contractions. I don't know the science behind it, but I think we have to be prepared to accept that people on the autistic spectrum have different tolerance to touch and also to pain.

I am sensitive to some smells, some brands of perfume are so painful on my nose it feels like razor blades. I also find I feel nauseous to certain smells. I am lucky as my husband is very patient about this, he knows I cannot tolerate a particular Calvin Klein product so he doesn't buy it anymore, or he used to put it on in the office, so I would not have to smell it until the end of the day when he had worn it in a bit!

I used to work with a girl who wore a perfume which hurt my nose; I asked her the brand and after a few weeks of tolerating it, I actually spoke to my boss about it. She asked the girl not to wear it as it affected people in the office, but sadly it backfired on me because the girl used to bully me after that. I learnt a lot from that experience, I now feel I can handle that sort of situation a bit better I wear high neck jumpers a lot and putting nose inside my own jumper does help, but that looks odd, so I open windows or I am lucky I can hold my breath a long time. If I am friendly with the person, I might speak to them personally about it, but I would find that very difficult. This is something to consider if you work with children, as some smells might be painful to them.

Tuning out!

Life is full of smells, sights and sounds which to someone on the autistic spectrum would be difficult to "tune out." I find it difficult to concentrate when I cannot tune sound out. I am involved in a number of voluntary projects. When I attend meetings I find it very distracting if a mobile phone rings or someone clicks their pen. I lose concentration very easily and it takes me some moments to get my thinking back to the meeting. This is more difficult when you are presenting or chairing the meeting. It is obvious if you lose concentration and you falter. If I am a passive listener, I can tune in and out of what is being said without affecting anyone else, but if you are contributing or expected to comment on what is said, you have to concentrate intently on everything. This is difficult enough as you have to tune out so many factors just to hear the words. In a group setting, you have to find who is speaking, watch their mouth to follow what they are saying, and if they move about that is another distraction. I find I am thinking – where are they going now? Are they going to trip on the cable? It is easy to lose track of what they are saying if you get distracted. Other distractions for me include the glare from lights on a screen, coffee arriving in the middle of a session, tea cups being stacked and cleared away, people whispering to each other, coughing, foot taping, paper rustling. The list will be different for other people, I have written about this as I think it might help others to be considerate as in meetings and in classrooms you cannot be sure who has a hidden disability and who might be excluded or prevented from accessing the information just because of overload of distractions or sensory overload.

To try and explain how it feels, and explain how the senses are overloaded, it would be like being in a flower shop where there are many smells and colours, then the language used might be like a foreign language depending on the accent of the person speaking, hand movements seem like sign language, jangling keys in pockets are like hearing shattering glass. The faces of the people are distracting, like having a tiger at one end of the table and a stick insect at the other. One with furry facial hair, the other slim and hair tied back. Then there is an overhead flickering of the lights which reminds you of a space ship and the papers on the table would seem like codes from a computer. I can concentrate and bring my thoughts into line, this is something that you learn as you get older, but I can imagine for some people that it is very difficult. If a child in a classroom is not motivated by the material or lesson, they might not bother to tune out the distractions and it might be more interesting to concentrate on their own sensory overload.

I work hard and concentrate on not being distracted by all the things going on. I try to follow what is being said, but I have written how it could

THE 'Q' FACTOR

be just to show how difficult it might be for someone on the autistic spectrum.

I find it a dilemma, do I ask people to refrain from clicking their pens as I cannot tune it out and it causes me to lose my train of thought? When a mobile phone goes once with a message, do I ask the person to put it to silent mode and please do not reply to the message as the clicking of the keys is also distracting? The noise of a pen being clicked over and over is so annoying to me. I'll try and explain why, I find I have to look for the source of the noise, that means I might lose my place if I am reading notes or overheads, once I have found the source of the noise, it feels like a cymbal in my head and takes the place of the speaking. That is the only thing I can hear and I have to watch the source of the noise, and the frustration level builds. Once it has stopped I can concentrate better. It is very difficult as people jangle keys in their pockets, they tap their foot, click pens, and all these noises are very distracting. You cannot tune life out; you do have to work at focusing on the important things like the talking. It is very difficult. I think that if I find it tricky, then a child must find it much harder and they might not be as motivated to work at it. It is easier to shut down and focus intently on your own body and retreat into a world of silence. Some people start to hum or rock to tune out the world around them and give their brain a comforting rhythm so that the overload doesn't hurt. It is more appealing to run through a particular interest, concentrate on something you like such as all your favourite DMU (Diesel Multiple Unit) trains or for me the current musical piece I am working on, rather than follow what is happening in the room with everyone else.

Irrational fears

I have irrational fears about travel. If I go on an aeroplane, I have to talk myself into it and spend the first moments on the plane praying that it won't crash. It's a very real fear, and I go through what I would do if we crash and if it would be better to crash over water, or land. In my mind I see picture of Tom Hanks in Castaway, that film brought my fear into the visual realm.

I am also afraid of rail travel and again I am scared the train will crash. For me, the fear is worse when I am travelling and not actually taking a part in the driving process. I am okay when I drive a car or ride a bike, but any public transport scares me. It is obviously something I deal with and have conquered, but it has not been easy.

I am also terrified of fire. I had a couple of incidents as a child which have left me very frightened. I was scared when a piece of smouldering coal shot out of the fire into my neck. I was only a baby, I do not remember the incident, but the scar reminds me and I am afraid around open fires. The other incident was when my Dad had one of his regular bonfires in the garden. He is a keen Do It Yourself enthusiast, so he often had waste to burn. He stacked the items into a pile and I was outside watching. I do not remember much except a burning paper sack was caught by a gust of wind and it seemed to chase me around the garden. It singed my hair and eye brows and I was terrified.

Malc knows how my fear regularly drives me to switch off electrical appliances. It is a major frustration for him as he plugs in his mobile phone to recharge it and I have switched off the charger at the plug. I think he now charges his electrical items at his work or in the garage! He also likes to leave things on standby, but I am afraid we will have an electrical fault. Living with Malcolm and having ME have really helped me live with my fears and deal with them because I wasn't physically in control anymore, I had to learn to trust someone else. I was too tired to walk around the house and turn things off; I had to rely on other people to do things for me. Because I had to prioritise my use of energy, turning off the electrical items became less important when I found it so difficult to get through the day.

When I lived in Canada for 1 year on a school exchange programme, I had to tackle my fear of fire as most homes have wood burning stoves. With one family, it was my job to light the stove in the den. I found it terrifying, but I managed it.

Malc would love an open fire, but luckily for me, we don't have a chimney. Ben is also a consideration, because he is weird around fire. He doesn't understand the danger at all. We don't light candles at all in our home unless it is someone's birthday or we have a very special occasion. Then we light candles and heavily supervise them. Ben dangles things in the flames and tries to chase the flame with his finger. It is frightening to watch, so we don't have fire around him at all.

Because of my own irrational fears, I can understand some of Ben's. For a long time, Ben was terrified of hand dryers, I think that is because of his hypersensitive hearing. He seems to hate certain sounds and will have a total crisis if it is not stopped. I used to dread going into MacDonald's toilets as someone would always wash their hands and the washers there are automatic, you get soap, then water then hot air, so it was bound to happen. His screams sound worse in a tiled confined area! Often I had to grab Ben, apologise as I squeezed past the person trying to wash their hands and rush out, I learnt to carry baby wipes and always wash my hands as soon as I arrive home! The hand dryer phobia continued for a few years, but gradually we could condition Ben to hand dryers, we found a public toilet with a very old fashioned hand dryer which didn't have the same loud rushing sound and it hardly dried your hands, but it helped us get Ben over his fear. He still doesn't like them and chooses not to use hand dryers, so I carry wipes and tissues. He tends now to come out of the toilet with soaking hands so the tissues are handy.

Another fear was of dogs. When Ben was 2 he was bounced in a park by someone's golden retriever, the owner knew his dog meant no harm but the fear lasted years. If we saw a dog ahead of us along the pavement, we had to cross the road and I would deal with Ben as he literally climbed up me to get away. He would cry, scream, kick and even try to scale a 6 ft fence in absolute terror. Then there would be splinters to deal with! (We have twice taken Ben to casualty with handfuls of splinters!) I am eternally grateful to friends who had a lovely dog called Jack. We took Ben to stay with them, and we all wondered how Ben would cope with Jack. When we arrived Jack was indoors, lying down and quiet. Because he was calm and not threatening, Ben could gradually get used to him. It took a week of intensive work; Ben patted Jack, then gave him some food, told Jack to sit, and eventually took Jack for a walk. By the end of our visit, poor Jack had so many walks each day by an enthusiastic Ben, that our friends told us when we left, he collapsed and slept for hours!

Ben was afraid of the things you put between shopping in the supermarket. The yellow triangle thing in Sainsbury's. It was okay in the Co-op as it was blue, but the yellow one was very scary. Supermarkets are difficult places for children on the autistic spectrum as they are large, noisy, and full of people and noise and the lighting is often very bright. All these sensations would be overwhelming and so for Ben, possibly the culmination of the visit to the supermarket when he was sitting in the trolley, was the yellow triangle

THE 'Q' FACTOR

waved too near him. Maybe it just caused sensory overload. We coped with shopping, but generally I tried to do it when Ben was at nursery or school. I did try to take him on a regular basis to get him used to it. I was lucky as our local Sainsbury's was next to the railway line. I used to park next to the railings where he could see trains. I timed our visits carefully when there would be lots of trains. Then I would take him in, telling him "trains later" he would chant "dains aater" all the way around the supermarket, with constant reassurance from me, we got through it. Then I could park him next to the railings and unload into the car. I knew Ben would not stray from the spot where he could see the tracks; it was brilliant as not only could you see the tracks, but you could see the trains going into the tunnel as well. So using Ben's passion, I could help him get over his fear of supermarkets. I still don't know about the yellow triangle, I was glad when Sainsbury's changed some of their colours and the yellow triangle has been replaced by orange I think.

So I know, fear is a real part of autism, but the fears can be managed. I don't know if you ever really conquer the fear, but you can have strategies to cope with it, so it does not dominate your life. New fears can crop up at any time, but you deal with them and learn how to manage them.

As well as fear of things, just as real is a fear of not fitting in or standing out for being too different.

I spend a great amount of time and energy worrying about what other people think about me. This might be irrational; if someone is upset or a bit abrupt. I wonder if I caused the problem. I worry about what to wear, what time to turn up. Should I start the conversation? Do you approach two people who are talking, stand silently beside them or try to join in? I still don't know the answers. I think sometimes I get it badly wrong and interrupt when I shouldn't and maybe I hover when I shouldn't. Decoding social situations is very difficult and getting things wrong is a real fear.

Detached emotional responses

My son finds it difficult to express his emotions. I know this because if you ask him if he feels upset, he pauses for a very long time and says "I suppose so." He may be displaying extreme behaviour such as shouting, screaming or hurting himself, but trying to find out what he is actually feeling is very difficult. He needs a lot of prompting and you cannot be sure that the feeling he describes or the situation he describes is current.

I found this out accidentally. My son was usually very stressed when he got home from his primary school. This is not surprising as the end of his school day was spent sitting in a hot taxi on the M25 in heavy traffic. The 22 mile journey could take up to 1 ½ hours. There were 2 other children in the taxi who went to the same school and a long suffering escort and of course the driver. We were very lucky as the 2 ladies who drove Ben were wonderful and we got to know them very well.

Ben would come in red faced (he would not remove his long sleeved sweatshirt, although he was obviously too hot). He would be very stressed and shout or scream. It would take a few moments to calm him down and we would begin the routine of a drink and something to eat watching his favourite video.

When he was calm, he might try to speak about what had upset him, this was very difficult as he found finding the right words difficult, but expressing the feeling or emotion was incredibly hard for him.

School is full of social situations to decode and relationships to cope with.
There were many other children who had similar difficulties to Ben at the school and unsurprisingly they would upset each other or "wind each other up." Finding out what had happened each day was very difficult, and we relied on the home school diary where messages between family and school were relayed.

One particular day, Ben was very upset and cried; the tears were in his eyes as he told me "Justin was naughty." This implied that the boy in his taxi had upset him that day, but I knew that was not the current situation as Justin had moved up to secondary school months before. Ben was using words from a previous occasion, he might have been feeling similar feelings of frustration or perhaps another child had done something which made him feel the same emotions. It is difficult to know for sure, but that moment told me that my son had difficulty with expressing himself due to his language difficulties and also difficulty identifying and naming his emotions.

It was good to have a clear example of this because I could refer to it later when teachers or classroom assistants were trying to make sense of what Ben was feeling. He could not always be relied upon to describe a current situation. Finding the words was so hard, that he found it easier to recount something from the past. In his way, I think he tries to express the feelings, the words describing the event represent the emotions to him but he might get specific details such as names wrong.

I think also that when Ben falls out with a particular child, he stores that moment in his memory and recalls it when a new situation occurs. He adds the wrong doing and layers it upon another in his mind. As in the film Rainman, Raymond lists injuries inflicted against him in a book, Ben lists them in his head and stores them for later. Crisis occurs or emotional overload when another small action is added to the list and the balance is weighed down too far. The final moment when crisis happens might be when only a small wrong is done against Ben, but his store of wrongs has reached capacity. He might lash out with an angry gesture or shout something at a child, but he does not usually strike them. There are some children who enjoy finding a way of annoying Ben, but they are probably not aware that he is filing all the moments away in his memory and the time will come when he reaches crisis point. I do not think some people with autism find it easy to cope with emotions. I am glad that so far Ben has not hurt another child, but if he reaches a point when he is overloaded with emotion, and frustration, he might.

I am very similar to Ben. I know this from my childhood and I am sure my husband will agree because in an argument or disagreement, I recall a situation he has long since forgotten, it has been stored away among the layers in my head.

Unlike Ben who usually manages to hold his emotions in at school, so that he doesn't lash out at another person, I have reached the point when I have lashed out against someone else. I was badly bullied by one girl in my primary school. She used to tease me and sometimes kicked me under the table if I had to sit near her. My Mum had been into school to speak to the teacher about the friction between the 2 of us in class so we were usually kept apart during lessons. The girl was very popular and I tried hard to get along with her. She was athletic and very good at sport – things which I am not! I envied her greatly as she always had friends to play with, she was popular and at the all important time when boys became interested in girls she received much attention. Some graffiti had been written in the girls' toilets about me and a particular boy, the teacher tried to find out who it was. It was totally untrue anyway but it was easy to find the culprit as the boys name had been misspelt. This was the moment of overload in my memory of wrongs she had inflicted. I challenged her to a fight after school. This was the first time I had ever stood up for myself and offered a challenge in this way. I wonder if the teachers knew about it, but turned a blind eye as this girl had made my school life such a misery for so many years.

I am not proud of the fact, but I really beat her up! My parents had told me not to fight, but my frustration and anger reached the point where I broke that particular rule. I had an older brother who had coached me in the art of "fisticuffs"! He had showed me that if you put your hand on someone's forehead, and stand back they can't reach you to hit you. I did that for a while and she flayed about in front of me. When she had tired herself out, I grabbed the hair at the scruff of her neck, which really hurts - I know this from personal experience from my brother! While I had her by the hair, I landed a left hook. I do not remember much else about the fight, but that was the moment she left me alone. I do not like to think that I had been in a fight and I am ashamed that I hurt her, but after that other kids did not bother me as much. It was the first time I had ever retaliated.

I found it very difficult to cope with the overload of emotion. I felt frustration and hurt after the constant teasing and name calling. The humiliation of having my name written in the toilets linked to a boy was as much as I could bear. Perhaps if I had tried to talk to someone about it, I might have coped better and not resorted to a fight.

Another similar moment occurred at home with my brother. He is 2 years older than me and knew very well how to tease and "wind me up". One day we were in the back garden and I told him I needed to go to the toilet. I ran in through the kitchen and upstairs. I had waited until I really needed to go, so to find my brother in the toilet before me, when he didn't even need to use it, was incredibly frustrating. He was only teasing as he knew it was quicker to run through the open patio doors into the house and he beat me up the stairs. I was so angry with him and this was one incident too many that I had stored away in my head. I experienced a moment when I saw red in my head and I hit my fist on the glass and it smashed!

I remember that incident often and it serves to remind me that I do have a volatile temper. Now I try to talk about my frustrations before they reach crisis or boiling point.

Sometimes I cannot identify the actual emotion, I know I feel major anger and I literally see red in my head. That is the moment I know to remove myself for time out. I think Ben is very similar; I try to monitor his stress levels and ensure he does not reach crisis point.

As anger and frustration are fairly easy emotions to identify and define, I find it is similar with sadness and grief. My son burst into tears when he saw a train crash on the news. He was not sad about the loss of life or the hurt people would feel, he was grief stricken that a 3 car DMU (Diesel Multiple Unit) was damaged and broken. He does get upset about an animal being hurt or if they get lost, but does not find it easy to understand other people's or his own emotions.

I find grief very difficult to cope with. I find I cry at all funerals I go to, whether I knew the person very well or if they were just an acquaintance. I try and blink back the tears. The way I cope is not to make eye contact with anyone else at the funeral. I do not look at the coffin and I can usually hold my feelings in check. I also cry at weddings, I do not know why. These are very happy occasions, so to feel the grief or feeling I know I experience at a funeral is very confusing. I try to hold back the tears at weddings, but I am sure I will cry at the weddings of my children.

The most traumatic funerals for me have been those of children. I cried when I remembered an image of the child, for myself at the loss of the small person in my memory but also for my son as they were children at his school. I then thought about the family members left without their child and that caused me the most grief. I found it very difficult if I saw the close family in tears or another friend crying. I would cry more at the image of that person's grief. I know the ache in my throat at funerals is the same ache I feel at sad films on the television. The degree of grief is much more intense at a funeral of someone very close to me, and I cannot cope with the intensity of the feeling. The sadness overwhelms me each time I feel it and it makes me cry.

Jealousy is another very difficult emotion to define and to express. I do not think my son can name jealousy as an emotion that he can identify, but I think he must have felt it at different times. He likes a particular girl at his school, she is very popular and at a recent ceilidh she is never short of partners. I think Ben felt jealous that other boys could ask her to dance or sit next to her and talk to her, but he just hovered around her but could not find the words to say.

As I have grown older, I think I can name and identify jealousy, but other emotions are still difficult. When a doctor asks me how I feel, I find it very difficult. A few years ago, I needed surgery for a gynaecological problem. I had to describe the pain I felt in my side. I found it very difficult to describe the pain. It just hurt a LOT! It helped when the Doctor asked if it was a burning pain or a stabbing pain, but I actually imagine if you are stabbed, the pain would feel like tearing or burning anyway. The operation revealed I had a ruptured appendix and a collection of very large ovarian cysts. (One was the size of a grapefruit). Knowing that text books describe the pain for as "some discomfort", I found it incredibly hard to identify the type of pain, and also where exactly it was located. I found it bizarre that I had also suffered a ruptured appendix as that was located on the

THE 'Q' FACTOR

opposite side of the abdomen to the cyst, but I could only describe feeling pain on the left!

Ben also finds it difficult to describe the intensity of pain and show exactly where he feels the sensation. We noticed he was very anxious and seemed more stressed than normal. He would get frustrated easily and seemed less able to cope with changes in his routines. When He started hitting his face we guessed that he might be in pain. He would hit his cheek repeatedly and try to rip his tooth out of his mouth. He cried out in anger. He was actually experiencing extreme toothache. After visits to the dentist and an extraction in hospital, the dentist showed me the teeth. They were so decayed; I cannot imagine the pain Ben must have experienced. He could not find the words to describe the pain, but his hitting his cheek was a way of communicating that he was in severe discomfort.

I know I can switch off and detach myself from pain because I remember an incident when I did just that when I was a small child at school. After an assembly we were leaving the hall class by class. I must have been in the infants as we were the first class to leave. My teacher led the line of pupils and opened the outer door. As I walked past I put my hand on the hinge and held the door frame. Pupils ahead of me opened the door wider and my little finger on my left hand was trapped in the gap between the door and the door frame. As people filed out of the hall, someone jammed the door open with a door stop, so I could not free my hand. At first the pain was excruciating but I tuned out of it and detached myself from the feeling. I was worried about being left behind but I could not move. I was left trapped until the last person had left the hall, by then my teacher had realised I was not in class and came to find me. When she saw me through the glass window in the door, she realised I was trapped. She removed the door stop, eased the door closed and as the gap widened, I could free my hand. I remember seeing my finger had ridges along it and the skin was hanging off in places. It took a few moments to feel pain, but as I looked at the finger, I can remember the visual picture triggered the pain. I had been able to detach myself from the feeling but then seeing the broken skin and blood, I felt an overwhelming wave of agony and pain. I was taken to sick bay and the finger was bandaged.

I enjoy acting a part, I think it sometimes helps me to cope with emotions I have buried or not been able to express. I recently went to a school days party and I dressed up as a rebellious secondary pupil. I found I took on the part of a girl I admired at school. She was not afraid of anyone and she always said what she thought without any fear of the consequences. I enjoyed being able to say rude things to people, show extreme emotions and behave like a spoiled teenager.   Luckily others at the party found it funny and enjoyed the character as much as I did. I felt bad after the party but it was fun and for the first time I had people asking if they could be my friend!

I have taken part in many amateur dramatic productions from serious to pantomime. At first I find the role difficult, but I usually base the character on someone else I have seen or copy another portrayal of the same character. It is fun to take on another character and react as they would react. I do not usually understand the emotions I am portraying, but I mimic someone else and how they express the emotions. I prefer to play a funny character and make people laugh, rather than make people cry. I find taking on another character through mimicry is a way of expressing emotions I have long since buried. It could be that well supervised drama classes in schools could be a good way of enabling children to express emotions and actually release some of the tension which can build up inside.

Detached emotional responses could be a reason why people with autism display unusual or untypical body language. I worry when I watch TV programmes when police speak about the body language of someone who is guilty. I understand that a person who is guilty might put their hand on their chin and cover their mouth; I do that most of the time. They might rub their ear lobes, my son does that just because he likes to do it, not because he feels guilty about something. I also do that frequently during a day as I like to check whether my ear rings are still in place. I think about my body language and because I have had comments made about the way I behave and about my intent staring, I try to copy what other people in a room are doing so that I do not stand out as different. This is something I have learned to do, but children with autism and young people might not have learned or been taught to do this.

Inappropriate or different body language and behaviour might cause real difficulties for a person with autism. If in a crowded place such as a train station, a Policeman called out "Stop!" to a person with autism, they might react in a very different way to a neurotypical person. Their reaction might be to run away as they feel threatened or frightened. The police man may well have had good reason to call to a person with autism. They might look suspicious just through their appearance. They might be avoiding eye contact, appear aloof and shifty because they like to stand first on one foot and then the other as that is a pattern of behaviour which might have a comforting effect or it might just be their normal behaviour. They will probably have a back pack which would contain their comforting possessions and wear a hat as they might not like wind or sound in their ears, they might even wear a balaclava as this is the best head covering if you have hypersensitivities. Alternatively, they might stand too close to someone else and stare at someone's pocket or bag just because they like the lines of stitching or because they are fascinated by zips. They might portray the image of a guilty person, but they are just different. If a person with autism were taken by the police for questioning because their behaviour seemed to be suspicious, it might be very difficult to really establish that the suspicion was only caused because the person acts in a way that is different to their neurotypcial peers. Similarly in schools people with autism are vulnerable as they can easily be blamed for things when their behaviour or body language suggested they were the guilty one.

Siblings

Lauren says –
"The good thing about my brother is that he is very kind, but the hard thing is that he can get very very very very stressed and I know he can't help it. It makes me feel upset. I hate it when he repeats the words on TV programmes, I hate it because you can't hear what anyone is saying. He also sings along to all the songs in a loud voice. It's very annoying. Even though we ask him to stop, he just carries on, and you have to watch his choice of programmes all the time too, it gets very boring."

Living with autism does bring stress to other family members. My husband and I talk to each other in code, if my son is in the room, he tunes into 1 word of what we are saying and you can never finish a conversation. My husband was talking to me about his day at work:

"it's a training issue"

That gets taken up immediately by Ben who starts on his favourite subject – TRAINS and he rattles off the "2 car DMUs are not as good as 3 car DMU" monologue.

We can't often have a proper conversation with each other, let alone other people! I find if we go out, I have Ben chuntering (affectionate term for

THE 'Q' FACTOR

monotonous questioning or repeating of
information heard many times before) in one ear
 "when are we going home?
we will never get home?
If I go to woollies, I can buy…."

When we are out Ben uses me as an interpreter,
he won't go and talk to anyone, but asks me what
they are saying or what they will do or stands next
to me and reels of his Christmas list in detail!

Siblings of autistic children have quite a lot to put
up with. They don't get much 1:1 as the child with
autism is so demanding. If I try and play a game
with Lauren, Ben joins in and takes over, it's like
the toddler stage when the child always seems to
want what another child is playing with, but with a
verbal monologue or running commentary of every
move!

Taking things literally

People with autism have difficulties with communication and language. This varies from person to person, but Ben has severe language difficulties. He was at a special school when we lived in England which specialises in speech and language. There he learnt to talk at the age of 7, and later learnt to read and write and communicate. Once he could understand more of the world around him, it became so much easier to explain things to him. We found out that we have to be very clear when we speak to him, say exactly what we mean and keep it simple.

We have had to really concentrate on what we say at home. Ill tell you a funny story – although it was not funny for Ben at the time.

He visited his Grandma, it was tea time and she needed to prepare the meal, Ben was very excited when she told him to "sit there for the present". He was still sitting there when it was time to go home, after tea and much later on, she couldn't understand why he didn't want to play. He was even really needing to go to the toilet, but he was waiting for the present which never came.

You've all seen the scene on Rainman when he is crossing the road and the sign says "stop" so he does – but that is in the middle of the road with traffic moving around him. Life is full of such

THE 'Q' FACTOR

Rainman moments for people with autism, the scene in the film demonstrates it very clearly.

Ben finds decoding sentences difficult; we use lots of visual clues for him at home. Reminders of routines, checklists, social stories, board maker pictures and symbols in the bathroom for the daily routines, charts in his bedroom for getting ready for the day. There are laminated charts and lists in every room in our house!

Sadly Ben experienced bereavement at a young age. One of his school friends died, and I found it very difficult to cope with him at that time. He could not make sense of it all and started causing difficulties in the taxi on his way to school, we thought it was because going to school made him think about this friend and the feelings he must have felt were very difficult for him to bear. So I sought advice from school and we I thought I was helping when I explained to him that his friend died in his sleep, so Ben might understand he did not feel pain, but after I had said that for weeks I could not get Ben to bed, and it was after much anguish that I figured what I had done was make him anxious of going to sleep. He was worried he might not wake up. So I used symbols beside his bed showing going to sleeping and waking up again and I started saying good night sleep well and see you in the morning. I still say that to him now.

Difficulties can also arise when people use figures of speech which are difficult for a person with autism to understand. You can learn what they mean, but each time the thing is said, it has to be processed and decoded into its literal meaning and then how it relates to the context.

For example, my mum told Ben one day she was going to spend a penny and his response was "what are you going to buy?"

My son got in trouble frequently at school for taking things literally. Once he was asked by a teacher
"is that **your** bag?"
My son's answer was just yes and he wondered why he got told off.
He did not understand the implied meaning, the teacher was really saying
"Is that your bag, if it is please move it as it is in the way"

Life is full of such circumstances and it is very confusing. It is like when we learn a foreign language and we learn text book sentences and phrases, language is full of common idioms and figures of speech and references which when you are learning a language at school you just don't have the time or understanding to learn. This is what it is like with autism.

As you grow older, you do learn to use figures of speech and understand the implied meanings but

THE 'Q' FACTOR

it is a learnt process, it is not innate which it seems to be with other people

Ben and I were doing some sewing. I was going to make a pair of pyjamas for his precious build a bear toy. I asked him to bring some clothes so I could use them to get the size right. He knew we were making clothes for the toy, but instead of bringing clothes for the teddy, he brought his own clothes. It made us laugh, but it was typical where Ben took my words literally, he brought clothes. He didn't understand my implied meaning or interpret the situation correctly.

Although I am aware that my son takes words literally, I sometimes get it wrong and cause him anxiety. Just before his 16th birthday my son was agitated. I thought this was due to the time of year as it was Christmas and we have family birthdays in December. The day before his birthday, my son had a conversation with me which made me realise that I had unduly caused him unnecessary worry and anxiety. Since he was 11 years old, Ben had been asking me when his voice would break. I would say "when you are about 16." I thought this generalised answer and the fact that he might have forgotten the question by the time he turned 16 would not cause him any worry. I was wrong! He told me that he was worried that he wouldn't be able to speak when he woke up on his birthday. He thought there would be pieces of his voice on his bedroom floor! We had a long talk about it and spent much of the day reassuring him. We told him that he would still be able to speak when he woke up and that it might yet still be some time before his voice broke. We explained that it was a process which did not hurt and did not happen at one time but that his tone would gradually deepen.

In spite of being aware of my son's difficulties, he still surprises me with his questioning and obvious anxiety about things which are routine and common place. Words and phrases sometimes confuse him rather than help him understand.

I am still all too aware that I take things too literally sometimes. I recently had some help from a neighbour who is an expert with computers and administration. He came to help me prepare a leaflet about access. He was showing me how to sequence the pages in the computer application and to help me understand; he took a piece of paper and tore it into small pieces. He smiled at me and said "I'm now going to make an elephant." Then he saw my confused expression, I was surprised that making an origami elephant could be relevant to a leaflet on outdoor access, but I carried on watching. Then my friend said "no I'm not going to make an elephant sorry it was a joke" he forgot that I take things literally did not understand his humour.

THE 'Q' FACTOR

Peoples awareness and judgements

Autism is a hidden disability. Ben looks "normal" so we often face judgement or criticism when trying to access services for people with disabilities. Surprisingly the disabled community is at times very judgemental too.

We have a blue badge as finding parking is important for people with autism. It might be a hidden disability, as the person with autism is often extremely mobile, but there are many reasons why people with autism need to use accessible parking spaces.

I applied for a blue badge after my son threw himself about in the back of the car when he saw the train station and I could not find a parking space. He saw the station symbol and could not understand why we were not stopping and going on a train. He injured himself badly and I was in danger of crashing the car. After that journey, I did 2 things, applied for a blue badge and also learnt routes which avoided train stations!

Where possible we use accessible parking bays as, you need the extra space around the vehicle to get children and belongings out of the car while hanging on to a limb of the child with autism! The accessible parking spaces are usually located near an entrance and hopefully without road or moving traffic between you and the entrance, because although children with autism are very mobile, they may have no road safety awareness. Although I always use the blue badge when I need to park with Ben, I have endured comments and glares from other blue badge holders as they just see a child who can walk and judge why I am parking in a precious accessible parking space.

People with autism find waiting in queues difficult – in fact waiting for anything is difficult. So going to a theme park where the day is spent in queues can by very stressful. At Legoland they have a wonderful policy that if you are visiting with a person with a disability you don not have to queue, so we took our family out and showed the pass to the ride operators and were allowed to join the ride at the exit. Other people in the queue were not happy about us doing this with a child who looks so "normal." When facing confrontation, I am not usually very good at replying to people who make comments, but Malcolm did better than me at Legoland after we had faced criticism at each ride, "
Do you want us to put our son in a tee shirt which says "yes I have autism" – just so you can feel better"?

Sadly sometimes even within the disabled community, hidden disabilities are misjudged or ignored.

I am passionate about speaking up for people with disabilities, especially those with autism as they sometimes get forgotten.

THE 'Q' FACTOR

From experience on the local Access Panel, I've heard the statement: "we have a ramp - so we are accessible," but access and Disability awareness goes beyond ramps.

To give you an example; improvements to the local bus service would make a huge difference to people. The local bus runs an excellent service, but accessing it is difficult. I have been working with Ben to enable him to use the local bus. This involved spending a few Saturday mornings in succession walking down our road to the main road and on to the bus stop. We had to cover everything from where to walk, where to cross the road safely, what to do if a car comes out of a drive, what to do if someone speaks to you or what to do if you see a cat or a dog on the other side? We are still working on how to cross the main road safely without of the help of the lolly pop lady.

Ben knows our local bus stop, and knows where to get off in Kirkwall, but getting home again is difficult. At the bus garage, the buses do not display numbers or destinations clearly, and it is also not clear when you are on the bus how you get it to stop! There are lots of buses which pull up at the Kirkwall bus garage, all blue, all looking similar. The driver might be different each time so you can't use that as a way of remembering which bus to get. It is very confusing for any visitor to the county, but especially to people with Autism.

Using the timetable is difficult enough, but how do you teach someone which bus they get when there are no numbers or destinations on them? I am sure most families expect that their 15 year old should easily be capable of travelling on their local town bus, but this is still an aim for the future, something we can't do just yet.

Ben is confident to walk to the local shop and home again now, so we are building some independence, but this has taken months of work – even now if he gets distracted he could be very vulnerable. I certainly would not let him walk on his own to a local shop if we lived anywhere other than Orkney!

Respite

I can't begin to tell you how valued and important this is! Respite is time given when your child with autism or additional needs is happily looked after – you can't put a price tag on it!

We have been lucky that we get a service called direct payments for our son. This funded time with a Personal Assistant gives Ben the opportunity to go out and take part in community activities supported by someone who understands his needs. During the time he is away, we can spend time with our other children. When my son is met after school and goes out for a couple of hours, I am so much more relaxed. My daughter can have a pal over for tea without worrying about how Ben will cope, or what he will say or do. We are lucky that we have good friends who have had him stay over night; I really love and appreciate that time. At home we can have junk food for tea, or a take away, without having to prepare something specifically for Ben and listen to him chuntering about how he doesn't like it. Although his alternative serving has already been prepared for him and his spaghetti hoops are already on the plate, he still complains very loudly about spicy food or "I can't eat that!" My daughter loves to light candles arranged on the table - we can't have any candles about in the house, as Ben likes to flick them and play dangling things into the flame.

I can relax, sit on the sofa and read my daughter a story, or watch a movie of her choice. This time makes her feel special and she loves it. Then when her brother comes home she finds she has missed him.

When it comes to bed time, I can actually watch the end of a TV programme, I can wear different pyjamas without the questions of what happened to the usual ones and am I moving house because the familiar ones are not around! I can have a glass of wine without being told it is bad for you or hear about the dangers of being an alcoholic. I can even take my glasses off and still be me, without my son running to find them. It disturbs him so much if I don't have them on as I don't look familiar without them.

The following morning, we can be spontaneous and take advantage of a lovely day and have an outing to the beach and kick the sand and sea without the moaning. We can get wet, throw stones for the dogs and not worry about finding them again!

Respite is so important. Sometimes we are just so tired from disturbed nights and stress during the day that when we get the opportunity of respite, we use the time to just sleep!

That's all without considering the planned outings like going to the pantomime or to watch Lauren in a concert. We have to try and find alternative arrangements and someone to care for Ben indoors as taking him really spoils the time. We have tried taking him to most things, but it becomes so stressful and he often spoils the event. Its not that we are mean and don't want our son to experience new things, we do them in moderation and when we feel both he and we can cope with it.

We got invited to Malcolm's family for Hogmanay and we took Lauren and Ben. We have a portable DVD player and set of headphones for Ben, the best purchase we ever made! He had his familiar story to watch, but he found the evening really hard. Once the movie had finished he got his coat on, zipped it up, packed his backpack and strode into the room and announced "its really time to go now!" My husband really wanted to see in the New Year, but I felt we should go as Ben was getting very close to crisis point. I still value our relatives and didn't want to put too much strain on the relationship or really have the young cousins see Ben at melt down stage. So we "quit while we were ahead" and left – it was 11.45pm so close to New Year, but it would have been a disaster to stay! This is not uncommon, living with an autistic person, things do revolve around them and how they are coping, so siblings put up with such a lot.

Partners and relationships are also under strain. Many marriages break down where there is a child with autism. The health of the main carer and other family members can really suffer. I am recovering from ME, I think my condition was caused by a number of different things, but stress doesn't help. Medics would tell me to limit the stress in my life and ask me what stress I had, when I explained that I have a son with autism, they would realise that was just something I had to get on with. Its not like a job; you can change a job, or move house away from stress, or even end a relationship with a partner who brings stress to your life, but you can't change your children! And actually I wouldn't want to. It's all about using strategies to cope.

My husband is very tolerant and patient, but he is under incredible pressure living with my son. So we really value the respite we get.

THE 'Q' FACTOR

Holidays

Holidays are usually happy times when a family relaxes together. Going on holiday with someone on the autistic spectrum however, brings many trials and challenges.

As a child I used to enjoy holidays, but my family stuck to a familiar formula. We used to pick a place which was fairly remote and quiet, therefore by holiday resort standards fairly boring. That suited us when we were young. As we became teenagers, we started to expect more from a holiday, but for most of young childhood, our holidays were pleasant experiences.

My parents would choose a self catering flat or bungalow, near the sea. That was the formula. My Mum would pack as much food and belongings as she could carry and then we would be off. We used to sit on the front door step wishing away the time and hoping my Dad would stay calm, but I expect the barrage of questions such as "are we nearly ready?" or "when are we going?" would annoy even the most tolerant person.

I used to spend most of the morning negotiating where we all sat in the car, as I knew one of my sisters would be travel sick. I still have little tolerance for vomit, so I tried my hardest to sit next to a window so I could stick my head out and try and forget or ignore the smell.

My father owned old cars and usually drove in a manner which would make even the most hardened stomachs lurch. I can remember praying as we pulled up at petrol stations – "please not kangaroo petrol!" He used to get so cross when he drove with kangaroo petrol, so we all hoped we would find a garage with the normal kind of petrol whatever that was! Even at a very young age, I used to take these expressions so literally.

The days on holiday were spent making huge packed lunches to feed the 7 of us and then off to the beach. It was official enjoyment at British best as we would be the only family on the beach sitting in deck chairs wearing shorts with cagoules and sun hats – hoping my Dad was right when he announced "its clearing up over there!" as opposed to the dreaded words "its clouding over!"

As a family we have found a formula which suits us. We bought an American style motorhome on Ebay! It is large enough to sleep 6 people, but the back, where a queen's size bed is usually located is referred to as "Benland." Home from home. Ben can pack his toys and belongings and it is familiar so that he thinks holidaying in the camper is truly the best holiday. He announced that he does not wish to go abroad anymore as it is too hot and it takes too long! (Both Ben and I suffer from prickly heat, so sunbathing in a crowded, expensive foreign resort, is not at all appealing).

THE 'Q' FACTOR

Whilst away, I am usually a little stressed until the morning routine has been accomplished and then I can enjoy my day. That entails getting 4 people showered and dressed and then feeding dogs and people and allowing excreting accordingly! Ben and I are similar in that we are organised and stick to putting things away after use. Malcolm and Lauren are similar in that they love to get things out and then leave them "handy for the next time." We are compatible as long as the tidiers stick to putting things in places where the others can find them.

Ben knows the campsites he prefers and we tend to stick to those. A preferred campsite is one with a shower block which is easy for him to use independently, and a small on-site shop as he loves to go and buy a pint of milk each day. Lauren and Ben love to ride their bikes around the site, so paved paths are best. That has become our favoured holiday.

I have already mentioned the need for visual timetables, so we have many discussions around what we are going to do each day. Those discussions are repeated, until adults are fed up with them, but we have to remind ourselves that routine is important. So we have to plan wet or dry activities for each day and have some concrete plans which we stick to whatever the weather. It is best if we write these routines and plans down for Ben.

We spent our most recent holiday in some severe
Aberdeen rain, but as Ben had brought his entire
brio collection back from a visit to his Dad, he was
amused inside the camper making creative train
layouts under the hanging wet weather gear and
around steaming drying dogs. Lauren tried to join
in, but Ben has a set way of playing with the
trains, which was not totally compatible with her
imaginative approach.

His Dad had originally packed the track and
engines in 2 bags for travel by plane, but although
we had more space in the camper, Ben would not
alter this packing in any way. We tried giving him a
larger holdall so that the entire brio collection
could be housed in 1 bag, but he still insisted on
putting the noisy battery operated bridge in his
back pack. This is just where it had travelled from
Gatwick to Aberdeen airport, where we met him to
start our family holiday. His collection of Hama
beads in 8 small coleslaw containers also travelled
up in the same bag, but some of the pots did not
survive the flight so there were loose beads
amongst the brio. At the end of each day, Malc
and I sorted the luggage into stowable dimensions
for the camper, but Ben re-sorted it to just the way
his Dad had packed it. We spent a fortnight tip
toeing around 2 bags trying desperately not to
disturb his backpack for fear of setting off the
bridge, as it was very loud. Malc even resorted to
removing the batteries, but this caused Ben more
stress as the following day he could not wait for

THE 'Q' FACTOR

Malc to have a cup of coffee before he wanted to make his train layout! We also made the mistake of putting some purple hama beads in with the yellow – then reconsidered this move when Ben announced daily he couldn't wait to get home, so he could re sort his Hama beads into the right colours!

Hot days on the beach or swimming in the river are great fun, but as soon as Ben dips a toe into the water, he asks "can I have a shower when we get back to the camper please?" This question is repeated until he has actually had the shower. I understand this is because he cannot stand the sensation of sand on his body. I am the same; I used to hate feeling sand and salt on my skin as a child. It is an annoying stage when you get dry after swimming in the sea, then you have to balance on towel and dry your feet and put them straight into shoes hoping you don't absorb any more sand on the walk to the car. I perfected the art, I would keep my feet bare until I reached the car and then sit and dry them and put on my shoes. The invention of beach shoes and rubber deck shoes has made things easier, but you still have to get that 1 annoying speck of sand off your feet! My Mum said I was a water baby on the beach, I think it was because I hated sand, and the water was a reprieve from the sensation of sand in your toes. It is also seriously annoying when your sisters get sand on your beach towel and why does sand end up in the sandwiches too?

Ben learnt to walk at 19 months old. He crawled from the age of 13 months until we went on holiday to Cornwall. I think that because he couldn't stand the feeling of sand between his fingers, so he stood up and walked around. We bought him the smallest wetsuit we could find, and he spent all day in the rock pools where he could rinse his fingers free from sand. When it was time to go, he would stand up and walk to the car and cry until he had a bath and was free of sand again.

Sand in the swimming trunks is also very annoying, Ben has a walk which I have grown to understand as the "I totally enjoyed the beach, but I really want to have a shower and get rid of this grit where the sun doesn't shine!"
People on the autistic spectrum have some totally infuriating habits but it is best to love them, or it could drive you to distraction.

Strategies

We all use different strategies to cope. Living with autism means you often have to use specific strategies to help get through the day. We use visual timetables, check lists, picture reminders and our latest invention – word cards. These are not a novel concept, but perhaps our use of them is new.

Meal times were fraught, all of us trying to speak at once and usually most people asking me questions. I found it exhausting and frustrating and it sometimes led to tears – not only mine! Knowing how important it is the have visual prompts; I had designed a "red card" for Ben. I have mentioned this else where. The red card was simply a small pocket sized card with the printed words "I need help." It was laminated and kept in Ben's coat pocket. It was designed for moments of crisis or confusion in the school playground when Ben couldn't find the words to say. With that thought in mind we created a set of cards which are kept in a basket on the dining table.

We agreed that we needed a visual prompt so that we all knew whose turn it was to speak. We thought about a toy microphone which each person could hold in turn when it was their time to talk. It was felt that this might be too distracting and mean that food would not be eaten; it is much more interesting fiddling with the on/off switch on a microphone or swinging it or twiddling the wires through fingers would be more appealing than eating food. We decided a card with the words "please listen, it's my turn to speak" would do the job. Once we started using the card, it became apparent that we needed many more cards with simple prompts written on them. We now have a basket full of multi coloured cards which are relevant to different family members. My personal favourite states: "I'm sorry, I'm too tired to speak." My daughter loves to select the blue card which states: "Relax." She uses this when it seems that Mum and Dad are getting cross with each other or they cant decide who forgot to collect the prescription from the chemist or buy the dog food. The cards are very good at diffusing a situation and save me a multitude of words. I can hold up relevant cards to 2 different people whilst at the same time speaking to my husband. This is a vast improvement on me trying to juggle responding to which 2 car DMU (Diesal Multiple Unit) is important, or listening to the date of the cello grade exam or figure who is going to take out the bin bags or walk the dogs! Whilst all the random chat is going on, you can guarantee that someone throws in a massive statement such as "I was bullied today." We've learnt the hard way that listening is important and that it is not possible to hear 3 people at once!

We have laminated table cards and also cards distributed about the house which state: "please wait, I will speak to you when I have finished on the phone." Although not to designer home standard, laminated visual prompts are certainly conversation starters. You would not see a red card stuck on most family window frames, but in our home, walls are actually educational and entertaining! Many visitors have asked about the cards and on noticing the one next to the phone, many have agreed that it really is "this seasons must have!"

I have prepared visual reminders to help my children get themselves ready for school. At the front door are sheets with photos of things they need for school on different days. It's a good way of building independence and it saves my voice and nerves! Many people agree they could do with such sheets in their homes so they remember car keys, change for parking meters, mobile phone or bags for the local supermarket!

Our strategies are both visual prompts and reminders but also agreement as a family that for anyone who needs it, time out is allowed. We have changed our spare room into a chill out zone. We have removed clutter and minimised the amount of furniture and distractions. We have put floor cushions around the room and have placed Christmas lights and lava lamps around so that they can be soothing when the day seems overwhelming. I have also got a posting box for Ben's angry sheets. The idea is that you write or type out what made you feel angry, then fold the sheet and post it in the box. Doing this helps get the frustration out and it helps leave the problems behind. We have a sheet in the room which states: "how angry do I feel?" there are options on the sheet from - very angry to a bit stressed, with a time allocation accordingly. Ben uses the room after school; he paces, flaps and rolls about on the floor on a big ball. It does help minimise stress. In the privacy and quiet of the room, he can carry out behaviours which help him feel calm – he is not the only person who uses the room, we all need space to relax and unwind!

Making choices is difficult for many people on the autistic spectrum. Limiting choices helps as often too much choice is just overwhelming. When the room is noisy or someone is listening to the radio, if Ben is trying to decide what to drink or eat, I often just show him the tin or bottle and give him a choice of 2. Rather than limiting him, this helps reduce his anxiety and gives him a sense of control. He is the one making the choice, I'm just helping by narrowing the options slightly. Sometimes spoken words are enough, but for a visual thinker, images are much more effective.

None of these techniques is really unique. I think in most homes where there is someone on the autistic spectrum the day is full of such strategies. I have included this section as a reminder of what works as sometimes going back to basic autism approaches, really helps get through the tough times.

Education

Finding the right school for a child with autism is difficult. We have been very fortunate with Ben as his early years were spent at a very good school. At 5 years old on starting school Ben did not speak, but by 7 the school had taught him how to communicate with words and sign language, and then with 1:1 and sometimes 2:1 input and coaching, reading and writing followed.

We have learned that we have had to be very proactive about school and do a lot of research ourselves. Not only do parents have to cope with the day to day issues of living with a child with autism but you have to campaign for the right school placement for your child and also for the support they need too.

This is constant and seems to be ongoing; at times, I have foolishly relaxed a little when we have a good placement for my son, and then all too soon difficulties arise which have to be dealt with.

Ben spent 1 ½ years at a nursery with 5 supported places for children who had speech and language difficulties. I found it quite upsetting when the nursery teacher took me to one side and introduced me to a new member of staff employed to support my son as they weren't able to manage him with the existing staffing ratio. This was in a place where support was much better than in an average nursery. There was a Nursery Teacher and 2 Senior Early Intervention Assistants and a Nursery Nurse and Speech Therapist. This was not sufficient so a person was employed to work specifically with Ben to ensure he was supported at all times.

I then realised I could not afford to assume anything with my son and his learning. He obviously needed more support than average. While he was undergoing the complicated and long Statementing process within the English Education system, I was busy trying to find an appropriate school. I had to do this independently and then try and persuade the Education Authority that the school I had found was the right one and hope they would pay the fees and transport my son there.

I found a lovely charity run I-can school which took children with speech and language difficulties. They showed me around and I felt I could imagine my son being there. At the end of the first visit, I sat and cried in the Head Teachers office. The school was wonderful but I was struggling with the fact that this was an environment where my son would fit in.

My visit included a tour around the school. I was impressed by the sense of calm in the school, even when we entered one class and the Teacher announced, "Sorry, Harry is on the roof again!" She quickly and calmly made a phone call and

THE 'Q' FACTOR

Harry was retrieved from his escape route. This must have happened regularly, because no one was worried. How Harry had negotiated the high and low double door handles on the 2 sets of doors and then limbered up the wire mesh fencing over the gate and up the fire escape onto the roof of the neighbouring building I could not imagine, but seemingly Harry was an "escaper."

I found it reassuring that nothing seemed too much for the school to manage. So after weeks of letter writing, meetings and finally assistance from my Member of Parliament, my son was enrolled at the school. I was fortunate to find a school that could accommodate my son's significant speech and language disorder, and cope with his autism.

When it came to the decision about secondary schooling, we found the task daunting. The schools which were suggested were over 300 miles away and Ben would have to attend as a boarding pupil. His primary school took children from all over the UK, but luckily we lived near enough for Ben to attend as a day pupil. He just had to endure 22 miles each way on the M25 in a taxi every day.

When it was time to consider secondary school options, my husband Malcolm and I visited schools recommended by the primary school team. We went to a school on the Isle of Wight, one in Nottingham and one in Kent. Whichever school we chose for Ben, we realised we would be faced with having a part time child. Ben would travel to school at the beginning of each term and he would have just 2 visits home and that would be the only time we saw Ben apart from school holidays. It was heartbreaking to consider this option for a child of 11.

At around the same time that we were thinking about secondary schools for Ben, my oldest son Nick was mugged and threatened at knife point. He was only 15 years old and travelling by bus to visit his Granny. This was a shock to all of us. It was clear that living in London, our sons were very vulnerable.

While considering these significant issues, we had a wonderful family holiday to Orkney where Malcolm's family live and we fell in love with the island. Fed up with long commutes to work and school, whingeing kids and hours spent in traffic just so we could pay an expensive mortgage, we decided to move to Orkney. We were fortunate that Malcolm found a job and we found a house which we loved. We were also impressed that the preferred option in Orkney is to accommodate children with additional support needs in their local community, so with the ideal of happy family life ahead of us, we moved up to the island.

We believed Ben would not have to go to a boarding school, and we hoped he could go to the school in our village. For the first time, I could have 2 children at the same school and Ben could have local friends. The secondary school for Nick was small with 400 pupils and it had a very good reputation both locally and nationally, so we felt our boys would benefit from a good education.

It was not that simple.

Ben could see his local school out of our window. He could see children walking to school and longed to go. However, despite dialogue with the Education Department in advance of our move and assurance that we could send him there; we were told at the last moment that the Educational Psychologist should see Ben first and do a full assessment of his needs. The comprehensive paperwork from his previous school which we had supplied in advance of our move was not adequate. We had submitted full copies of all Individual education plans (IEP), the Statement of Educational Needs and updates, notes and transcripts of reviews and reports from all the professionals who worked with Ben. This included reports from Speech Therapists, Occupational Therapists, Physiotherapists, Paediatrician, Social Worker, School Nurse, Teacher, Head teacher Educational Psychologist and Crossroads coordinator.

The Head Teacher had looked at the paper work and I guess had thought that on paper Ben looked very challenging. He did explain to me that he was worried that local school could not support

Ben adequately and that the special provision on the island might be more appropriate.

So Ben went to the small special school where he stayed for 18 turbulent months. I have great admiration for all the staff who work at the school, but at the time, the needs of the individual pupils were so diverse, that it was very challenging. Academically, Ben did not progress very well. He was so unhappy that we actually noticed some regression. His speech deteriorated and he became much more volatile. He even became aggressive at school. In his early school years we found with Ben that he would usually hold his emotions in check at school, but he would let rip at home. This is fairly common with some children on the autistic spectrum and fairly similar to my own school experiences.

For a time, Ben's behaviour changed; usually he was accommodating at compliant at school, but we noticed that he had become violent and aggressive at school. He even threw tables about in frustration and directed his anger and frustrations at staff. These were the actions of a very unhappy child and I knew I had to help him and make some changes.

Ben wanted to go to his local school. He had got to know some of the children at our local church and he wanted to be with them at school. He loved to sit with them on Sundays and he resented knowing that he was the only one who did not go to the local school. He found their sophisticated behaviour difficult to understand and was often behind in understanding what was expected of him, but he had become an incredible mimic and would watch the other children and mirror their behaviour. For the first time, he felt part of a group. He did not always stand out as different. You could even lose him in a group of children playing, but watch him closely and you could see him watching another child and copying their every move and expression. He is such a good mimic that in a crowd he does not appear any different to any of the other children. He and I are similar, we watch what is going on around us and copy what other people do, this makes you seem to fit in and appear normal. There are however sometimes when it is obvious that he is just copying others and not understanding what is going on around him. There was a week at church when most of the other children were away on a school trip; Ben sat at the front of the church where the children usually sat. The Minister announced the hymn and he said "we will remain seated for this one." Ben was the only person who stood throughout the whole hymn. There were no other children around him that he could copy; he was the only person in the front row so he could not see that everyone else was sitting down. I was in agony in my seat further back. I thought, do I walk to the front and tell him to sit down and draw even more attention to him not understanding what was said? Doing that would also make him feel embarrassed as he would realise that everyone else was sitting down. I decided to leave him standing; at least then he would not feel any discomfort and he was totally unaware that he was the only person on standing.

We Knew Ben was unhappy at the special school and he constantly asked why he couldn't go to his local school like the kids he knew in our local area, so we campaigned to get a place for him there. He had 2 hours a week as part of a shared placement, which he enjoyed so much. Monday and Thursday were shared placement days and they were the only days Ben went to school without a fight. Shared placements are used in Orkney when a child goes to the special school out with their local catchment area. The child spends most of the school week at the special school and spends 1 or 2 hours per week at the local school so that they spend time with a local peer group. I thought that a shared placement sounded a very good idea but we found it was a frustrating experience for our son. Difficulties can arise in that the child falls between 2 schools. They are on the school record in one school only, so unless they have a very understanding and proactive school office at the shared placement, they only get letters and included in school events at the main placement. We found that Ben did not always get information from the local school only from the special school. We found that we missed information about local activities as the special school did not always get included in letters about extra curricular activities and Ben would not get a letter from the local school as he was not counted on the school roll. I think it takes a lot of effort from the parents to ensure that their child is included fully in both schools.

In the local mainstream school during some of the shared placement, Ben did not even have a desk or a peg allocated to him. At the open evening, we were invited in to meet the teacher, but there was not a tray or any work for us to look at. This was disappointing. It may be that the school had not experienced a shared placement before. We felt that the Education Department should provide advice or a model for the school to draw upon, so that families are not expected to educate the local school about what is expected. We assumed that at least a child like ours should have the same seat in the class room, so that he would know what was expected and where he could go when he arrived. It was a supply teacher who was responsible at the time, and perhaps she had not worked with shared placements previously – or with pupils on the autistic spectrum.

We had to be in constant communication with both schools. There was one occasion when we had to write an assertive letter to the acting Head Teacher as she advised us that as the class room assistant was on leave so the shared placement could not happen for a week. We were very disappointed and challenged this as it was an experience our son looked forward to so much. We requested that the school considered supply cover so that our son could still benefit from the shared placement, we were lucky that this was agreed and our son did get to continue with the placement that week. Sadly the Education Authority do not have a budget for support staff supply cover, so this was an expense for the local school and I can understand their reluctance to spend money which is always needed for other resources and budgets. It was easier and cheaper to assume that Ben would miss the shared placement the day the classroom assistant was to be absent.

As I've already stated, and as many other families who have a child with an autistic spectrum disorder are aware, as parents you have to stay proactive and keep focused on your child's education. Ben showed us that he was unhappy at the special school and I started thinking that perhaps inclusion in mainstream was the way forward.

The Education department considered our request and we were so lucky that our local school took Ben on a full time basis and not just in a shared placement. He spent a happy year in a mainstream P7 class and joined in all the activities of the school. It was successful because of the hard work, careful planning and commitment of the Learning Support Teacher and the Classroom Assistant. As a family we are very grateful to them because they worked so hard and gave Ben a successful mainstream experience.

THE 'Q' FACTOR

This was the best social time for Ben, when he attended the local school. He got to walk to school for the first time. Following weeks of heavy shadowing, coaching and support when we worked on where to cross the road safely, told Ben what to do if a car started reversing out of a drive, what to do if someone calls you across the road, what to do if you see a dog, cat, bird or something different to the norm. Gradually over months Ben could walk part of the route on his own without an adult minder, but with a carefully selected P7 friend who lived nearby.

There were many firsts during the year at the local school. Ben sang his first solo in a school concert; took part in local school fund raising events; went carol singing in the village; went on his first residential school trip; had a school photo with his sister and wore the same uniform as everyone else in the village for the first time ever. He also had his first ever party with school friends and even took part in a youth club sleep over - with help and support from people in the local church.

For the first time, local children would turn up at the house, knock on the door and ask for Ben. We think it was something to do with our wonderful trampoline, but without a doubt, this was the best social time for our son. Now there are 6 other trampolines in the village!

As school systems are different in Scotland, Ben benefited from an extra year at primary school as children move to secondary school a year later than they do in English schools. When it came to choosing a secondary school at age 12, we were hoping our son could go to the same school as his brother and with his peer group from our local school. It seemed this was not possible for Ben. We visited both schools and spoke to the Head Teacher of the smaller local school, but he told us that he did not feel that his school could cope with our son. This was because of Ben's language difficulties; the Head felt that the teachers would not be able to differentiate the curriculum. As the Head seemed so negative about our son, we did not have the heart to persist with our application. We took the advice of the professionals and enrolled Ben in the larger of the 2 secondary schools on the island, the place which had the special provision for pupils with additional needs.

We had got to know some of the staff at the school and we know how hard they work. Ben's Guidance Teacher is a friend of ours and a Deacon at our church so we felt confident that he would do all he could to support Ben and we hoped things would be okay. Ben moved to the new school with the support of the Classroom Assistant who worked with him 1:1 at the primary school. A lot of effort was put into the transition, but despite the hard work and efforts of individual members of staff, sadly the decision was made to reduce the support and by the end of 2nd year,

THE 'Q' FACTOR

Ben was in classes without any support and he was struggling. We are very grateful to the Teachers and Classroom Assistants, who have really tried to help support Ben, but decisions were made at a senior level and reducing support had a negative impact on our son.

While writing this, my son has had to cope with bullying, anxiety and stress at school on a daily basis. Some of the situations he has to cope with are unacceptable but we have felt unable to do anything about it.

Last summer when the school timetable changed my son got locked in the gym changing room for a whole lesson. This was very distressing and he now has a real deep seated fear of locked doors. The incident happened because Ben was not supported. Forward planning is something people with autism find difficult. Ben went to his first lesson following the new timetable, but did not plan ahead and carry his gym kit with him so he could go straight on to PE. This meant he had to walk back to collect his PE kit from his peg, and then go to the lesson. By the time he arrived at the changing room, all the other pupils had already changed and were in the gym. A member of staff let Ben into the changing room at one end, without checking that the other end of the changing room was open. It had already been locked. Ben was extremely traumatised by the incident and even 1 year later; he still worries if doors are locked.

The school doors are now locked during the school day. We understand the need for this security measure, but Ben finds it very upsetting and spends much time each day worrying if he will actually ever be let out of school. It would have helped if parents had been advised of the new security measures. If we were aware of the changes, we could have spent time talking to Ben and preparing him for what would happen. We could have given him strategies to cope and taught him the procedure for asking to leave school early if you need to go to an appointment and also what to do at the end of the school day. Most mainstream children would not worry about the installation of the security lock, but extra thought and planning should have been in place to support any pupil who would have had difficulties understanding the changes.

Recently Ben's phobia about locked doors was made worse as some pupils decided to lock him and another pupil with additional support needs in one of the classrooms. This is the actual place where pupils are encouraged to go and where a member of staff should always be on duty so that pupils should feel safe and supported! It so happened that the member of staff who is usually in that suite of rooms was off sick, but there was no one else there to replace her to ensure that the pupils were supported.

Ben comes home from school anxious and frustrated most days, some are worst than others.

THE 'Q' FACTOR

It can take days for him to speak about what has happened. I have to spend a great amount of time coaxing information and help him tell me all the confusions in his head. If he has had a very bad day, he paces up and down and I can see the tears in his eyes as he fights to stay composed. To stop himself crying, he pulls his lower eyelids down so that you can see the red of his eyes and he rubs the actual eyeball. The sensation and emotion of crying is overwhelming and the lump in your throat and the heat of tears is unpleasant. I get a sore neck from trying to hold back emotion and I think Ben makes his eyes very sore with his method of stopping his tears.

The incidents where the doors were locked have been very traumatic for Ben. He is afraid that he will be shut in and he will never be let out. It is not a rational fear, but it is a real fear to him. It would be helpful if time was allowed for teachers to help children cope and progress through such fears and worries about school life. If anxiety levels are too high, a person cannot learn so I personally think it would be very helpful if pupils were helped through such incidents and the confusions of social situations at break and lunch times. But this is not on the national curriculum so schools must find it difficult to allow timetable time and resources to teach such things.

Because of his level of difficulty in some areas, Ben is in the bottom group for most subjects. This is no fault of his own and he wants to work. He has to cope with the disruptive behaviour of disaffected pupils who basically do not want to be at school and who would prefer to annoy class mates and their teacher rather than do any work.

In some Scottish Secondary schools, the level of support for pupils like Ben has been reduced greatly. This is following recommendations by HMIe. It is thought that 1:1 support does not help pupils gain independence. Although this might be the case for some pupils, I do not think that it is helpful for some pupils with autism, as support is needed to help them understand and access the curriculum and *all* other aspects of school life.

Some pupils like Ben might be quiet in class, they might be cooperative and compliant, but I do not think the education they receive in mainstream classes is always meaningful. We watched a national TV programme filmed at Orkneys biggest secondary school with interest. Ben was in many of the episodes. We were very concerned when we saw our son in mainstream English. He was sitting fidgeting at the front, wearing a large set of head phones. The other class members had all been preparing a talk about an animal which they were to present to the class. With support, there is no reason why Ben could not have done this activity. I would have helped him with material as we live in a house with 5 animals and we also foster cats for the local Cat Protection group. Ben is very interested in animals and could have focused on his own pet or the work he does helping with the foster cats. While watching the TV programme we asked him what he was doing at that time in the class and he said "that is when I was listening to Charlie and the chocolate factory on a story tape!"

I do not think this is accessing the curriculum on any level!

I recently attended a Conference on Autism and Education at Aberdeen University. By luck and poor planning on my part, I ended up in a workshop entitled the right training. I had assumed it might help make decisions for Ben beyond school, but it turned out to be discussing training for teachers! I felt out of place but I was able to make some points which they had not considered. I said that I felt inclusion in mainstream worked better in primary schools but at secondary level the subject teachers didn't always have time to differentiate the curriculum or time to learn about all the differing needs of the pupils in the classroom. Without support from trained classroom assistants, the inclusive approach could not work. The workshop facilitator asked how many teachers in the room were secondary mainstream subject teachers – there were none! That is my point.

I would like to make a controversial point that I think it might be useful for Education Department officers to go back into classrooms to see what it is like for people with additional needs and also to experience and appreciate the pressure that teachers and school staff are under! If Education Department decision makers and budget controllers could spend a day in the support for learning departments in a school – they might realise that their budgets need to account for supply cover for support staff, time for mainstream teachers to differentiate their lessons and classroom supply cover for teachers to attend relevant training. It would also be useful to speak to the pupils; those in classes with disaffected pupils and also pupils with additional support needs. They would give an interesting view on how inclusion affects the learning of all pupils. But I am not a professional educator.

Secondary school education in mainstream schools focuses on exams. So much of the curriculum and school life is centred on qualifications. If like Ben, due to ability you cannot access the level required to take and pass exams, then it can be very demoralising to continually read reports with X and fail written in them. We do not show Ben his reports as he gets so upset by them. He feels he works hard and puts in so much effort, but he reads comments and statements which do not reflect that.
Achievements of pupils without the academic ability to gain passes in national tests and exams should still be celebrated. When exams, prelims or mock exams are going on in school, support staff are redeployed to scribe and support pupils in their exams. Other pupils with additional needs

still need the ongoing support in their classes; I feel strongly that additional supply staff should be found to help during these times.

My own school experience is probably not uncommon. I attended the local primary school and then went on to the all girls secondary school. I decided to go to a single sex school as my experience of boys was that they bullied me, generally I was the one who had snow balls hurled at them or whose school bag was thrown down the stairs.

I have described some of my memories of primary school in an earlier section, but an overwhelming memory is that I often felt totally confused about what was going on around me. I remember the difficulties I had making friends and that play times were incredibly stressful for me. I remember one particular day that I was standing outside next to the water fountain. This must have been a day when I was discovered in the cloakroom and was turned outside to play. But I did not know how to play with the other children. It was a total mystery to me. I remember a girl called Lavonia. She had lovely long blonde hair. That day; she came over and beat me up as I just stood there. I do not really know what provoked her. As I try and recall the incident, I can only imagine that she thought I was staring at her, perhaps I was. I remember I was fascinated by her hair and I wished I was popular like she was. I did not know how to fight back and I remember the pounding fists on my arms. She had 2 other girls with her and they laughed at my lack of self defence or retaliation. I had been told by my parents not to fight and that in the bible it says not to fight but to turn the other cheek. That is what I did. I was upset that I had been in a fight, but confused and frustrated as I did not even know what had caused the attack. I remember being very wary of Lavonia after that moment, I always kept my eye on her if we were in assembly just so I could see whether she was going to beat me up again.

My strategy was probably not a good one. It might have been my staring which offended her. I know that now schools do work with pupils who have difficulties with social interaction, they can teach them how to approach other children and how to moderate their behaviour so that they do not draw attention to themselves or provoke others. So hopefully they wont get into fights like I did without understanding why.

There is also now more understanding in schools about the benefits of visual approaches such as visual timetables and clear visual routines. I remember being so confused about what I was expected to do next. In the early 70s the trend was for choice and open plan group work. This is a nightmare for someone on the autistic spectrum. I preferred the classrooms where the desks faced the front in rows and where we stuck to a timetable. In the infants, the day was flexible and we could move around the class from one activity to another. I used to always stick to hand writing which is what I enjoyed doing. I did not like the Wendy house, and I did not know what the story corner was for unless the teacher was there and we all sat together and listened to a story. I can remember being slightly slower than some pupils at picking up writing skills. We had story boards with words to pick and use for a story. I could read the words without any difficulty, but I had problems thinking of a story.

I am also aware that at school I found verbal instructions difficult. It was so much easier to follow a lesson when the teacher used the black board. People on the autistic spectrum do usually have difficulties with language, so allowing processing time is very important and also using visual clues. I attended a National Autistic Society course recently and was told about the 6 second rule. When we say something to a child, if they do not respond straight away, it is tempting to flower or complicate the language further which only adds to the confusion. Instead we should allow processing time and wait for a response without complicating language further.

For example:

"Put your books on my desk when you have finished"

Further complicated by:

"If you put your books on my desk quietly and in an orderly manner then we can all go out to play."

The person with the language difficulty will be still processing the first sentence and may be stuck on the first few words. Further language is confusing and frustrating.

Vulnerability

Ben often comes home from school very upset. This is sometimes because children with autism are easy targets for bullying and taunts from other children.

We have even visited the police station to report an incident involving a child from his school. It happened during a weekend when Ben was with a carer. She helped us understand his anxiety about the incident. Ben was hounded around a local supermarket by the girl and she terrified him. She told him she would kill him, and because he takes things literally, he believed her. He tried to run away and she chased him, this only made him more anxious and frightened. This incident occurred while he was supported by a carer, the situation would have been much worse if he was on his own. He would have been so much more vulnerable.

Ben is also vulnerable as he is an easy target for manipulation. He has been set up by other children who are more devious and able to manipulate than he is. They may tell him to say something to another child or to an adult. The remark will probably be hurtful and will get Ben into trouble and it might also greatly upset the other person. But he does what he is asked to do, because he wants to please the "friend" who has asked him. It is not difficult to imagine the potential for trouble.

My own child hood memories are full of such incidents. Even my own brother would set me up to get in trouble. On one occasion he told me to take a badge from another child's coat. He liked it and wanted it, but after I took it I wouldn't give it to him. He then told our parents and I was in big trouble! My brother's favourite game was target practice – with me as the target! Or we used to "play tying up." He would always tie me up first, and I would have to sit tied up until my Dad came home from work and released me! I never got to tie up my brother as I could not untie myself in time!

Because people with autism take things literally and they are generally honest, they can be very trusting and therefore an easy target. Trying to please friends or desperate to fit in they might be inadvertently led into dangerous or criminal activity.

I would also like to mention here the potential danger of the internet for people with autism. There are many forums, games and chat rooms which are easy to use and people with autism might prefer computer contact rather than face to face contact. Computer contact is preferable as you don't have to worry about interpreting facial expressions or people's emotions.

A person with ASD might not understand implied meanings and could be easily manipulated. They might not understand that the person they are corresponding with might not actually be who they say they are.

As parents and professionals I think we need to be very aware about this. I know of a young person who was manipulated by someone in an internet game site for children. Posing as a young person, in reality they were actually a 37 year old wife and mother. The young person was groomed and manipulated into meeting the person – and led into a very adult world. I have also heard of young people who have been persuaded to give out personal information. They have been duped into sending explicit photographs, video or web cam footage of themselves and their friends. They might have been persuaded to give out passwords which in turn allowed access to secure information on their computer. I think young people on the autistic spectrum are potentially more vulnerable as they are more trusting.

Home School

Some of the difficulties we have experienced as a family are not uncommon, so it is easy to understand why many families opt to home school their child. Following a very traumatic bullying incident I withdrew my son from school. This decision was not taken lightly as home schooling is very challenging and I am not convinced that I am very good at delivering it! My son had been very unhappy for months. I was in dialogue with the Education Department and the school, but the reality for my son was that support in the classroom was not happening so his self confidence and self esteem were taking a battering. Feeling you do not understand is not a pleasant experience, this was happening in lessons on a daily basis and my son was not able to do the work. His school report was a disappointing reflection that some of the subject teachers did not understand his needs.

I only had to home school my son for a short time, but it was an exhausting experience. I had to keep motivating him to do the smallest tasks and each project had to be broken down into easy understandable and manageable stages. I can identify with his difficulties in understanding a whole task and feeling overwhelmed by a project as a whole. It is necessary to break things down and take a task one step at a time.

THE 'Q' FACTOR

Each household task became a learning opportunity. I had to continue with the things I do around the home, so I used the tasks to teach my son. I called laundry and cleaning Home Economics. We planned the menu for the day and went shopping - each stage was an opportunity for learning. We looked at the ingredients of food and discussed what foods are healthy. I know these are things he had already learned at school, but some of the learning in the classroom he finds difficult to transfer to real life situations. As I discussed things with my son, I could see more and more just how his understanding limited his ability to carry out many every tasks. We watched the Kim and Aggie "How Clean is your house" and it helped him understand the need for cleaning and hygiene in the home. When his bedroom or his sisters becomes too cluttered, I only have to mention the programme and he asks "they are not coming here are they?" It is a great motivator for my children to keep their rooms tidy. Ben doesn't understand that Kim and Aggie are invited to a home but he worries that if our house is not tidy, they might just turn up on the doorstep!

Taking the animals to the vet for routine injections was an opportunity to discuss vaccinations and diseases and taking precautions for animals so that they do not become ill. I tried to discuss the need for human inoculations too, but my son found transferring the learning at the vet to a human scenario too difficult.

We spent time learning how to send messages on the computer using email. I was trying to make his time at home useful and meaningful and teach him skills he could use in life beyond school. Following a period of such intense anxiety and stress however, much of the time was spent relaxing and allowing the opportunity to discuss things which had happened at school and to unravel some of the frustrations and worries in my sons head.

I enjoyed seeing my son more relaxed and calmer as he did not have to face so many difficult social situations but I was very aware that isolated learning would not be good long term. As I had to cope at school and although I hated it, I had to continue and learn lessons about social situations and about people, similarly my son would have to return to school and progress his learning.

Before he returned however, I did have opportunities to discuss his needs with school and some of the processionals involved in his life. We had invaluable assistance from Advocacy Orkney. By this time I was feeling very overwhelmed and exhausted by the situation. The Advocate helped voice concerns on our behalf. Having her at meetings was reassuring as I was worried that my emotions or difficulties expressing myself might have got in the way of my sons needs being met.

THE 'Q' FACTOR

My son returned to school and joined a different class. He went into a more supported environment and started a new timetable. He continued with 2 mainstream lessons and the rest of the time he was placed with other pupils with additional needs. We discussed the return to school and although he wanted to continue "home school" he understood that we could only do this for a short time while the teachers sorted out a new timetable for him. I gave my son choices, he could either return to school and continue his existing timetable with more support in the mainstream classes or he could re join the pupils he knew from the special school in a different timetable. He made his own choice.

Work

School days are hard, but life beyond school is very worrying. The transition from education into the world of work is a difficult one for many people, but for people on the autistic spectrum it brings many challenges.

Finding the right job is difficult. Thinking about a career is difficult; it is an abstract process as you haven't got the necessary experience to make that leap from what a job is like in brochures or advertisements to what it is actually like in every day terms. If I could not imagine what it would be like then I know it must be a concept my son finds difficult. I was offered careers advice at school and it was suggested that I should be a teacher. I asked if I could study typing and commerce as I thought I might enjoy working in an office, but I was told I could not do that as I was "too bright!"

I drifted from one job to another and I found work difficult. I found personnel suited me as I could work alone and I was happy keeping records. I could recite the entire staff names, dates of birth and national insurance numbers as I spent so much time processing and recording the information. When I first start a job, I find the first day very stressful. There are so many new situations and concerns; where do you hang your coat, what is expected of you in your role, what do people do at lunch time, will you fit in socially?

THE 'Q' FACTOR

Understanding and accepting office etiquette is challenging. When I look back over my work history, I cringe with embarrassment, but I think some of my mistakes could be made by any one on the autistic spectrum. There are more strategies and supports available now, but unless the condition is understood by employer and colleagues, then there are bound to be misunderstandings. I have learnt strategies over the years, but when I first worked in an office, I made mistakes and was ostracised by colleagues. In my first permanent job, I was not given a written job description, so I did not really know what tasks I was responsible for. I did process all work put in my in tray as was expected, but I did not answer the phone as I find phone work challenging and I was trying to concentrate on the work on my desk. I did not understand that as I was at the reception desk, I should greet all visitors and also answer all phone calls. This did not go down well with the other girls in my department. I thought my priority should be the typing given to me by colleagues who were insistent that I should do their work first. It became difficult as many of the tasks were deemed priority. I did not have a superior who prioritised my work for me so I was burdened by the pressure of demanding colleagues. I am aware that I believe most things I am told, so when someone tells you that their work is the most important, you have no reason to doubt them.

I found the volume of work overwhelming and I got frustrated by my mistakes, but I did master the typing and gradually got on with the tasks and learnt how to do work the way particular people liked it. I wrote copious notes which my colleagues found amusing, but I needed to refer to the notes each time I carried out a task. I had lists of information of abbreviations, wrote out phone numbers so I had them to hand when members of the public requested the information. Some of my idiosyncrancies have been adopted by others over the years, but mostly I was an object of fun.

When new to an office, it is difficult to know whether you make tea and coffee for all colleagues every time you make one and I did not understand the rule of buying cakes on a special occasion for many years. Understanding the language and humour of an office also takes effort. In a sales office, I began to understand that smutty humour was acceptable, layered with sexual innuendo and that most people used expletives in every sentence! It took me many years to adopt the language of my colleagues and I was always teased as being different.

I found it very difficult when someone would look over my shoulder at what I was doing. With personnel work, I had a good excuse to turn my computer away so that no one could see and my work station was set up in an office where I was on my own with my back to the wall so I could see anyone approach. I find it very worrying if someone hovers behind me, it is too unpredictable. My boss stood behind me when he wanted to see some information and I froze. I could not remember how to look up the file name and I was struggling. In the end I said, "I am too nervous with you standing there", his reply was "that's a relief; I thought I'd hired an idiot!"

I was very fortunate that he was a very patient Manager and he trusted me to work on my own and knew I would get the job done. He asked me to take on payroll in addition to personnel. I tried to avoid it, as I was so worried that my poor maths skills would make it too difficult. It was a new task, and the thought of any new task is very overwhelming. He said he thought I was the perfect person to do the payroll as my approach was methodical and consistent; it was just what was required.

I was totally honest in my work, even when I made mistakes. I could not sit quiet and hide them or blame them on someone else. I would hold my hand up and admit it was me. Once I put the wrong toner in the printer and it would not work. The office relied on the printer and I was goaded into doing it by my colleagues. They would not take the risk themselves as they guessed it would not work if you put photocopier toner in a printer. As I was desperate to be liked and to please my colleagues, I went ahead and it broke the printer. I was very worried that I would lose my job. The Manager wanted to know who had done such a stupid deed and the supervisor tried to diffuse the situation and did not blame me. I was worried that the supervisor would get into trouble for my mistake so I went to see the Manager and confessed. I felt awful but I had to do it. People with autistic spectrum disorder do generally find it difficult to be dishonest.

I was careful with my time keeping. That does not mean that I was always punctual as there were inevitably days when I was late due to traffic or my son's taxi to take him to school was delayed. But I would always make up the time I owed to the company. If necessary I would work later or I would take work home. When I was fairly new in one job, I was working after my set hours and a colleague said "Trude, you are beyond your sell by!" I think they were surprised that I bothered to make up the time as that morning I was 5 minutes late.

In most jobs, if you proved yourself by working hard and obeying rules then you would usually get on okay, but I learnt that being diligent is not always popular with colleagues. It might be accepted by Management or in fact taken for granted by them that you would always work your hours and get the job done, but colleagues might be resentful. Some people like to play the system and get longer breaks, delay work or spend too much time on cigarette breaks I did not see the point of this. I was in work to do a job, so that is what I would do. I would feel guilty if I had to take a personal phone call and I would make a conscious effort to make up any time spent on personal matters. In some jobs I had, this was not the office culture, so I was bullied in the work place.

I think I am an easy target and I found office humour difficult to understand at first. There were the usual sexual innuendos and I was always the one who was set up for those. When I was working in personnel I found I had a good reason to separate myself from my colleagues as the work was confidential. That made it easer for me as I was happy working alone.

Common to many people on the autistic spectrum, I am a perfectionist. I also have a fear of failing. I think we are our own worst critics in that if we do something wrong; we will be the ones to condemn ourselves for it. Other people at work seem to have the ability to laugh about mistakes or jokes made about them. I find that very difficult. I do not understand teasing as I take words too literally and I think it can not be a joke. One person I worked with found that I was easy to manipulate. She would give extra work to me and took pleasure of humiliating me in front of others. If I made a mistake, she would laugh about it with colleagues, but I did not do the same to her.

I found it difficult to compete with office banter and when taking phone calls for others I would dial the person's telephone extension and speak to them on the phone rather than shout across the office above the noise. This was thought to be quaint and I was teased about it. Another observation was that I called people by their name rather than by the popular derogatory label or name they might be given by staff. I found it impossible to say "that annoying git from…" or "the fat ugly guy from stationery!" I genuinely thought that the person might hear. I usually called people Mr or Mrs rather than first names, I don't really know why, it has been a source of amusement to others in places where I have worked.

I find it very difficult to use office jargon and the latest phrases. One such sentence I find difficult is "buy into it." Do you have to actually spend money to make a commitment to a process? I think it means support something or agree with a way of working, but I am not sure I really understand the full meaning. It seems to take me longer than other people to fully understand and use some of the accepted phrases. I am afraid I might use them incorrectly and I have to decode the words before I can use the phrase and this often interrupts my thought process. I found "brain storming or thought shower" sessions very difficult as I could not get the image of rain alongside a cross section of a brain out of my mind.

In an office, you are often expected to distort the truth so that you can cover the mistakes of others or explain why they are late for a meeting. I found it very difficult to field phone calls for my boss. If he did not want to speak to someone, it was easy for others to say "he is in a meeting" when I knew that actually he was not. I used to say "he is not available" but that was not always as successful as the excuses used by my colleagues. Persistent callers could usually get round me so I had to learn phrases to use. I struggled to say words that were not literally true, but adopted expressions as "he is not at his desk" as an acceptable way of deflecting a persistent unwelcome caller. I wrote lists of phrases to use to begin and end phone calls. I copied language used by colleagues and built up a directory of expressions. For some tasks I actually wrote entire scripts. I would practice these scripts when I was driving to work, and I would go through possible scenarios in my head in advance of a conversation. I envy people who can leave their work behind them at the end of a day, how ever small or trivial the tasks, I do not find it easy to switch off from what I am expected to do during a working day.

I do not find working in groups very easy and I have come to the conclusion that I am not cut out for committee work. I find I get very frustrated as I try to communicate a point. It seems that people do not understand what I really mean. I used to think it was the other person, but more and more as I have blamed others for not getting my point, I have begun to assume actually I might not be making the point effectively. Having decided that committee work is not one of my strengths I feel a sense of relief. I find it very difficult to assimilate information in meetings, I need paperwork in advance and generally this does not happen.

Trudy Marwick

Invariably some reports or materials are presented at a meeting which you are expected to read and work on then and there. The level of frustration builds as this occurs to the point where I am so overloaded by frustration that I cannot really concentrate on what is being said anyway. It is also very difficult to concentrate on just the spoken word with no visual clues as people debate issues around the table. I am really not good at committees!

In my work environment I like a clearly defined work space. I prefer to work with my back to the wall so I can see anyone who might approach and I like to place where people are in the office. I find it difficult to ignore the movements of others so I tend to keep track of where other people are in the office. This minimises the possibility of surprise. I get frustrated if people sit in my personal work space as they might move things and I am used to my things in certain order. I find it very annoying if people borrow office stationery and then don't replace it. When I worked in an office, I don't think I was popular as I am one of those people who labels staplers and hole punches! Where others welcome the break and the chance for interaction with colleagues, I find it annoying as I just want to get the job done and not spend time searching for the elusive stapler! I know I am very rigid in my thinking, but I have my reasons for this; I need a certain type of pen as being left handed, my writing gets smudged if I use roller pens. I guard my preferred pens and my husbands knows that borrowing the pen in my filo fax and not returning it gets me very annoyed. I have become aware that my habits might be very annoying to others, so I now try to leave pens around where others need them, for example by the telephone or calendar. I check these repeatedly during the day as it is very annoying if they get lost.

I spent a great amount of time writing task lists in my work and ticking things off as I had done them. I found the day too overwhelming if I did not plan my work. It was easier to see things written down and I find it very satisfying ticking them off. I probably spent too much time working on checklist and task lists but I found I could not work effectively without them. I did get very frustrated if my plans were interrupted. Sometimes I did find it very difficult to prioritise tasks so I would ask my Manager if he would tell me what work he needed me to complete first. This structure helped me get through the day without feeling I could not cope with the workload. When I was processing the payroll I would ask my colleagues to minimise interruptions - this was one of the very few times they would comply with this request.

Since my diagnosis I have been very worried that I am not good at communicating and I think I am guilty of email overloading people. I am so worried about not passing on information that over compensate and send messages to people as I think of things. What I should do is plan carefully think things through and then combine the smaller points into one bigger message. I am not sure what people prefer. As thoughts enter my head, I have to say them or act on them rather than plan and think things through. Forward planning is not one of my strengths.

I want to fit in an office environment, but I have found it very difficult socially. Lunch times are difficult as I want to be alone and walk out in the fresh air. I find it frustrating if people try to arrange to meet me or want to walk with me as I need to be alone and have time for my thoughts to slow into neutral. I used to use the lunch hour to go to the gym or for a run, but often someone would want to come along. I plan my hour rigidly and someone else would invariably slow down my routine. I even tried to join a lunch time running club but found running at the pace of other people too frustrating so I stopped going. I would make my route cross that of the club runners so that I could meet up with them along the way, but I prefer to be alone.

Work social events were difficult. These occasions just made me more aware of my differences and I label myself socially inept. I was happiest if I was organising them, then I felt I had a role and it kept me busy. I used my children as an excuse not to attend too many work events and the annual Christmas do was an event I did not always enjoy. People would make you drink at their pace, and I really can not keep up with seasoned socialites. I would end up making a fool of myself and then be the butt of more jokes for the next month. Where others seem to enjoy the attention, I hate being a source of amusement or conversation matter for others.

It has been difficult finding work experience placements for my son. He started a placement in one of the local music shops, he really enjoyed the 2 hours a week he spent there. Sadly the placement was too high maintenance for the member of staff. My son needed constant supervision and reminding not to play with materials but to stay on task. She had to communicate the same instructions to my son each week. She had to keep him on task and motivate him and doing this meant she could not concentrate on her own work, so he had to stop going. He was quite upset and I learnt lessons from that placement.

My son is nearly 16 and like many other parents, I would like him to have a Saturday job or a way of earning some money. Finding him a successful job seems daunting as he has such high support needs. I started asking him to take some responsibility for tasks in the home. To earn some additional pocket money, he started doing the dusting each weekend. This was a trial as I had to spend 2 hours with him, reminding him what to do, keeping him on task and making sure he remembered which things to dust. I could understand why the work experience placement broke down.

It became clear that my son needed a lot of structure and very clear instructions. In order to work independently, he needed a sequence of visual instructions and clear targets of what was expected of him. I devised a set of visual aids to help him. As I know that visual clues are essential for my son, I photographed each thing I wanted him to dust and sequenced them on a sheet. I wrote the amount of money earned for each set of pictures and included a photo of the tools for the job at the start. I gave clear instructions about when the work could be done and what was expected before he earned the money. We learned many lessons perfecting the sheets but my son has been using them successfully for some months now. They help him work on his own and get the work done.

When a new work experience placement was offered for my son, I spent a great amount of time with the supervisor as she was keen to help get the support right for Ben so he could work as independently as possible. We devised a set of sheets for him to use. He was to help at a local church lunch club. This involved setting and clearing tables and serving customers. There were many barriers we had to overcome to make the placement successful. We spent many hours photographing the steps involved in each task. This included sequences of photographs showing things such as the cupboard where tables were kept, photographs of how to erect the table, photographs of the products used to clean the tables and where they were kept to the stages involved in laying a table. We ensured that we showed hands actually putting knives and forks on the table, so that it was clear how the cutlery arrived in each place setting and that it was not done by mystery or magic. We also photographed some place settings which were incorrect and used these as training tools so we could discuss "what is wrong in this picture?" The visual approach worked and my son has spent some months helping successfully at the lunch club. The feed back has been positive and he has not been a hindrance to other staff, but his contribution has been valued and he looks forward to going each month. He takes his folder of sequenced photographs and his apron and walks independently to his work experience. It is wonderful to have found a successful strategy and system of support which suits my son. It was time consuming setting up the sequences of photographs, but I use this approach for other tasks. The only tools needed to implement this strategy are a digital camera, printer and glue! Photographing actual items is more effective than clip art using other symbols. People on the autistic spectrum are literal thinkers and so a generalised image might not represent the actual object which means something to them.

Faith

On his website Daniel Tammet writes about his faith.

"I think many people are surprised to hear that I believe in God and that I am a Christian. I think this is because many assume that autism and belief in God are somehow incompatible. In fact other autistic writers, such as Temple Grandin, have written about their own spiritual beliefs and practices".

Being brought up in a church going family; I was used to going to church on Sundays and could recite hymns or passages from the bible. As a young child I was brought up hearing about God but it wasn't until I was a teenager that I believed the words for myself.

I have always believed the bible was true, and I had no difficulty understanding that God is our Creator and that he has an awesome plan for us. I feel I am lucky as I take the bible as true and believe what I read. I do not feel the need to debate huge sections of text to test if they are credible or right, I accept the writing as words from God. I am sure even writing this might stir up challenges and comments from others who dispute the teaching and writing in the bible, but even at my most rebellious moments, I have always believed there is a creator God who loves me and part of his plan for me and anyone else who believes in Him is that he sent his only Son to take on the sins of the world and bridge the gap between Creator and creation.

I am lucky that mostly believing and faith comes relatively easy to me, I believe in the Trinity and the concepts in the bible. I find some of the language difficult to interpret and I am sure I miss a huge amount of implied meanings. I am glad that Ministers and other more experienced folk can make sense of it all.

There are mysteries in the bible and the stories but to me I guess I keep it simple. I believe God is real and he answers my prayers. I find it is awesome that we are allowed to know God as a personal Father. I think I am lucky that I was brought up hearing words from the bible and that I had the opportunity to ask Jesus into my life personally.

I have learnt a great deal from my son about what faith really is. Ben was recently baptised. He became a Christian last summer after we had a talk at home about what knowing Jesus really means. Ben has been going to church since he was born. His father takes him and recently here in Orkney we attend the local Baptist church.

Like me, when Ben heard the words "Jesus loves you" he accepted them as true. He speaks of his faith and openly tells people he is a Christian. When I was trying to complicate things by assuming that my son might have some difficulty understanding what the bible says about baptism, my son assured me that he did understand. When the minister visited and asked him why he thought he should be baptised. He said "it says it in the bible, and I am a Christian".

My son chose this song for his baptism service:

"Jesus loves me this I know
For the bible tells me so
Little ones to Him belong
They are weak but He is strong

Yes Jesus loves me
Yes Jesus loves me
Yes Jesus loves me
The bible tells me so"

I don't think I can argue with that.

Being part of our local Baptist church I have found what it truly means to be part of a Christian family. There is total acceptance for people as they are. You feel that you are welcome and you are welcome to bring differences and real life with you.

We have a small group locally which meets each week. As a family we have found real friendship and acceptance there. It was at a small group meeting that I first told people that I have Aspergers Syndrome. It was the week it was my turn to try and lead the bible study – something I find particularly challenging as I do not feel my bible knowledge is deep enough and I know my weakness in interpreting what other people say so I might miss really important things. I thought I should admit my difficulties at the beginning of the evening, so that people could accept my limitations and help me out by joining in and saying what they felt about the passage.

I don't usually say much at all during bible study as I am worried that my understanding is not necessarily right and I might totally misunderstand the bible passage. It always means something personally to me, but it might not be relevant to anyone else. I feel quite inadequate about sharing what I think bible passages mean.

Being part of a church is much more than meetings. I have found not only acceptance in the church but also meaningful support. That has been both practical and spiritual. That means you get help from others when you need it practically and also when you need advice about your faith, or a person to listen to your worries or problems. When I was ill with ME at my worst, it was the actions of local Christians which meant such a lot to me. Friends came and took the dog for a walk for me and a neighbour collected my daughter from nursery. This practical help I think spoke more about their faith than attendance of a Sunday service.

I have heard some people say that people use faith or belonging to a church as a crutch. I take that to mean, something to help them walk or stop them falling down. Perhaps that's part of it, there have been times when things have been tough and faith has stopped me falling down. It is maybe seen as a form of weakness of character that you cannot struggle through tough situations without having faith to depend on. When I am confused about people and how they react to me, or I feel they are not there to be a support when you need them, I know I can depend on acceptance from God.

I know I get it wrong sometimes and say something that is not particularly sensitive to someone else's needs or situation. It might cause someone hurt or pain, but I am so glad that I don't have to worry about getting it wrong with God. You can talk to him and actually he does understand the implied meanings completely.

I'm not perfect and sometimes I do still anguish over why I am different and why I struggle with friendships and relationships. Then I remember that Jesus went through every single emotion that we did. He was "despised, rejected, a man of sorrows;" any of the feelings we struggle with sometimes, but yet Jesus actually didn't deserve any of it like we do.

I come to the conclusion that it doesn't matter if you are different. A real church is an accepting church. My son goes to church carrying soft toys which are sometimes elaborately dressed up. He may be wearing a sweatshirt with toothpaste on it or cat fur where he just grabbed the cat as we were leaving. His collar is usually lopsided and his hood half tucked into his coat collar. He is always accepted and welcomed at church. It is understood that he finds loud noise difficult and he may shout out or react differently to other people at something unexpected. When the Minister goes through the congregation to ask someone a question, he doesn't leave Ben out as his answer is usually unpredictable, but if Ben puts up his hand, he is included and valued.

At the beginning of the morning, Ben and Lauren love to stand on the balcony and throw toys down, it is of course very amusing if the toy lands somewhere inappropriate such as the collection plate or on someone as they walk in. This behaviour is not reprimanded or stopped but instead, the person usually throws the toy back up.

At his youth group recently, they were talking about what real love is. When he was asked the question, what is love? He answered "Kirkwall Baptist Church."

Sometimes fewer words actually say more.

The Ups and downs

This has been all too serious and sobering, but I feel it important to understand that living with autism, or obviously with any child with additional support needs can be very challenging. Most of what I have written could apply to other families who live with someone who has a disability or additional support needs; and of course they also have additional stresses and pressures which we don't. Life has his challenges for any family, but perhaps those people with autism bring another dimension to family life.

Strengths and magic moments

People with autism have many strengths. As I have already written, my son has perfect pitch which is a real gift. He has an amazing ability to retain facts and can tell you anything about his favourite subject – Diesel multiple units (DMUs).

When you live with some one who has difficulty accessing many situations and finds participating in normal events quite a challenge, when they do that that step and make the effort to join in, it brings a magic moment which is irreplaceable.

I have many magic moments and memories which I cherish. I will always remember the time Ben sang a solo at a concert in his local school play. Not only was he in costume, taking part in a dramatic production, but at the end of the play, he led the school in a rendition of "walking in the air"

THE 'Q' FACTOR

the song from the snow man. With the right coaching, I am sure he could have made a recording to equal Aled Jones, but I didn't matter that it was not as musically perfect; to me it was a magic moment and much more of an achievement.

I will also cherish the memory of my son's first sentence at the age of 7. I was at my mum's house and we were busy cooking the dinner. Ben was amusing himself with lego in the next room. He was very busy but after much concentration, he came into the kitchen and said "I have made a house" it was a phrase lifted out of a story which I read him most evenings. The small boy in the story says "I have made a crane", it was an amazing moment as Ben had taken this phrase, used it appropriately and changed the right word to make it fit the moment. He had made a lovely model house. My mum and I nearly dropped the dinner as this was the first sentence we had ever heard him say.

I will also clearly remember the first time he showed empathy. My daughter Lauren had very bad chicken pox and her face was covered in the distinctive spots. She was lying in my bed with me and Ben came home from school. He burst into the room full of life, stopped dead in his tracks when he saw her and came over with a worried look on his face. He sat next to her, put his head to one side, put his hand on her knee and said "oh dear." Those 2 words summed up all the things we were all feeling at that moment.

I will also remember a similar understanding and use of empathy when I was upset after our cat had to be euthanized. I was a bit emotional and Ben came over to me, put his hand on mine and said "ahhh, are you cold enough?" The words weren't quite right, but the sentiment was clearly there. It was magical.

Some Ups - Funnies

I'd like to end with some of the ups and downs of living with autism, and talk about them in a humorous way, as even the downs have their funny side – when they are past anyway.

Sometimes the tough times are very hard when you are going through them, but after a while, you can look back and smile about some memories. Ben was sent a beautiful Gund beaver from close friends in Canada. He had it since he was 2 months old and it became his very special cuddly toy. He took beaver everywhere and wouldn't sleep without him. Because he couldn't say the "v" sound very well, beaver was affectionately known as "Beeber." We had a few close shaves as we nearly lost Beeber while on a shopping trip and he was left behind in a shopping centre once but he was found the same day and returned to Ben. However, when Ben was 3½, Beeber was left on a bus and we didn't find him.

THE 'Q' FACTOR

It was a particularly traumatic trip that day. I had
managed to haul Ben away from his favourite
video and persuade them that a trip on the bus to
the local toy shop and MacDonald's for tea would
be fun. It was time to buy new shoes, always a
very traumatic event. Ben hated having his feet
measured, in fact he hated having his shoes taken
off and he hated having to try on and then wear
new shoes. Ben was not very happy about the
outing, although I told him we were going on a bus
to a toy shop. I would broach the subject of new
shoes when we had got to the shop. It was a
wonderful "Mothercare world" where you could
buy shoes and then look at the toys all under one
roof, all the time not letting Ben out of sight as he
could so easily set off the automatic doors and
escape into the car park – but that is another
story.

Ben cried along the road to the bus stop. We saw
a bus pulling away as we approached the bus stop
so that did not help. The next bus that came
stopped and I folded the buggy ready to get on.
The bus driver insisted that he would not give me
change from a £10 note, so I decided to go home
and get some coins and wait for another bus. Ben
could not understand this at all. On reflection if I
had realised what was going to happen, I wish I
had just given the money and lost forgotten about
the £8 change. I could not afford to be so
frivolous with money. Ben cried all the way back
to the house and then cried all the way to the bus
stop again. We sang his favourite songs but he

was fed up. The next bus came and we got on.
We went upstairs to keep my older son amused as
he preferred being on the top deck. I don't know if
it was the sheer exhaustion or the fact that I was
worried about hauling uncooperative Ben down
the winding stairs on a moving bus, while keeping
an eye on his brother that made me forget to
check that we had Beeber. We did not have
Beeber. He was left sitting on the top deck of the
number 140 bus to Hayes and Harlington.

For what seemed weeks, Ben cried every night for
Beeber. Eventually, I managed to get him to
understand that Beeber was not coming back. I
laugh at the memory now, as it is amusing but at
the time it was very difficult. Ben stood against
the wall, he put his hands behind his back, took
deep breathes and said "shit!" I could not correct
him; it was totally appropriate use of language,
said with expression and at the right time. Now,
the memory makes me smile, but that day, there
were not many smiles in our home.

We have since got a new Beeber, by the wonder
of Ebay. It has taken 12 years, but searching the
World Wide Web paid off. I hunted in charity
shops, my friends in Canada kindly tried to get an
identical beaver, but the gund version was not
available. They sent a beautiful substitute beaver
who arrived in a parcel in very fast time. It was a
true mercy mission, finding Beeber. The smaller
beaver was adopted by Ben and loved almost as
much, but in his heart I think he really missed

THE 'Q' FACTOR

Beeber. For many years he could not even look at any photo which included Beeber without shedding a tear.

I searched for a gund beaver for many years. One day, I did my usual search on Ebay and found the exact beaver staring out of the photo. I bid straight away. I would have paid £100 for him, but gladly I didn't have to as I was the only bidder. When the auction closed, I emailed the seller as I was so thrilled to find a true replacement for our Beeber. She emailed back delighted that he was going to a good home and told me that this was a charity auction and the money raised was going to help children with autism!

When the parcel arrived, I could hardly contain my excitement. Beeber was lovingly wrapped in a tissue and laid in a box fastened by a button. I put it on Ben's place mat on our kitchen table, and waited. When the school bus arrived, Ben rushed in as usual, ready to start pacing and complaining about his day. He noticed the parcel immediately, dropped his school bag and coat on the floor and rushed to open it. I watched his expression. He hugged the beaver, and exclaimed, "Beeber, where have you been!" Then he blinked the tears away and said, "I think someone has washed him." The new beaver was so soft and in perfect condition, Beeber was loved and had a washed in feel.

There was no pacing and complaining about school that day. Ben decided that Beeber was to stay in his bedroom and not go on outings as he really didn't want to lose him again.

Other funnies…

We bought a new toilet seat from a local store to brighten up the bathroom. The one we chose has dolphins on the seat and lid. Ben helped Malcolm install it, but later that day, I saw him dancing about in the hall and I asked him what was wrong.

"Someone has taken the toilet."

He could not figure out how to use the new toilet seat. He could only see the dolphins and had no idea that they were decorations on the toilet seat. His visual recognition only saw the pictures of dolphins and he could not see the toilet as a whole anymore. I had to show him that it was still a toilet and show him how the new seat and lid worked.

I can see around corners:

People with autism find it difficult to see things from another person's point of view. So if they can see something, then surely you can see it too.   I first saw this in action when Ben had a conversation with his granny on the phone. He was pointing at his train track, and saying "that train over there" he believed she could really see it too although she was 800 miles away.

THE 'Q' FACTOR

This can have advantages as well as disadvantages. For example, I can tell Ben his picture is very good from 2 rooms away. I can see around corners and tell him that I can see that picture on the internet of the 2 car DMU southwest trains in southern livery too! Sadly, my talent for this does not work with Malc when he asks me if his tie matches his shirt. I hear him from another room "I'm not Ben!" So I do have to get up and go and actually have a look!

<u>Downs and scary moments</u>

There are ups and downs living with any child, but living with someone with autism can bring unexpected challenges. My worst moment ever was when I took my son on the waltzer ride at a theme park **once** – this was definitely a once only ride! He wanted to go on it, but when it started he decided he wanted to get off, so he did! He slid under the safety bar and lunged to get out; I just had an ankle in my hand! It was so scary. His flaying hands were so near the wheels under the spinning car. I hung on to his ankle for what seemed ages, whilst waving madly at the ride operator with my one free hand. After waving in vain for what seemed an eternity, I then hung on to the ankle with both hands to ensure I had a firm grip. Luckily for me, an onlooker saw what was happening and got help to stop the ride. I got off and had to continue as normal. What I wanted to do was shout at the ride operator, but that would not have helped Ben, he was very upset and I was very shaken but we went on our way with the promise of ice cream to calm both our nerves!

Ben does have difficulty differentiating between fact and fantasy. After watching the film "Harry Potter and the Chamber of secrets", I found Ben pinning the cat down and shining the torch into her eyes. I released the cat and asked Ben what he was doing? He told me he was trying to make the cat "petrified" like Mrs Norris the tabby cat in the film! He genuinely believed that if she looked into the torch, she would go rigid like Mrs Norris and then he could make her better using "Mandrake roots" as in the film. Thinking ahead and forward planning is also a difficulty for people on the autistic spectrum. This is shown here too as Ben had obviously not thought things through; he had not got a supply of Mandrake roots in advance, ready to make the remedy potion for his cat!

Difficulty with fact and fantasy does cause other problems – how do you explain to a child that writing a letter to Father Christmas asking for an invisibility cloak might not mean you actually get one for Christmas? Then, if you did get one, how would you explain that it did not work! That same year, the Harry Potter interest continued, and Ben wanted a wand for Christmas so he could make his sister "be good!" This would have been another tricky one!

On a visit to a prospective new school – Ben asked the head teacher if they have a "chokie" at

THE 'Q' FACTOR

the school. The Head Teacher looked at me a little confused. Ben had only been to a small special school in Surrey, his understanding of school life was limited to that experience. This was his first visit to a local school and I think he thought it might be like the one portrayed in the Roald Dahl story Matilda! Sometimes fiction or fantasy can help make sense of the world, but there are times when it makes it more confusing.

Some of the downs experienced living with autism are to do with the need for routine. When I had just given birth to Ben's sister (a home birth to minimise disruption for Ben), I had to get out of bed almost straight away to process Ben for school. It is normal routine, so it had to be done! When he came home that evening I had to get up to bath him as normal, it was exhausting, but necessary.

Living with the routines of people on the autism spectrum can be physically exhausting. As I have mentioned, even on Christmas day we have to do the same routine which is hard on the other family members. You end up trying to maintain "Benland" while giving the other family members an enjoyable Christmas too. Christmas is a happy family time, but to people on the autistic spectrum it can be one of the most challenging times of year as there is so much disruption to routine. There are school plays to rehearse, songs which you only sing at Christmas, parties, Christmas meals, gifts and cards to write and receive decorations to disrupt school and home, and different food to eat.

We have some bad memories or "downs" that are to do with food. Or being precise – food fads! Ben likes Marmite sandwiches, but he doesn't just mildly like them, he is passionate about them. He even ran away when we went to a picnic recently as I forgot to bring his marmite sandwiches! If we go out for a meal, we have to plan Ben's meal carefully and if necessary pack a lunch box for him! You can't be spontaneous and just decide to go out for lunch on Sunday or go and grab a coffee in town without considering how we can sell the idea to Ben first, pack his alternative menu and bring something for him to do while sitting in the restaurant. Going for a meal is actually boring for some children, and I think more so for children on the autistic spectrum. Our other 2 children love to go out for a meal, but Ben fidgets, fiddles with cutlery and anything on the table, clinks the glasses with his tea spoon as they do in the Harry Potter films, makes his own version of a glass harmonica, makes flying origami planes and rocks on his chair. These things in isolation might be funny when a toddler does them, and may raise a smile the first time, but the novelty has certainly worn off as he does them every time we go anywhere for a meal.

I also have some memories which are embarrassing. Things I'd really rather forget as the situation could have been dangerous for Ben or others! I have one such memory when I was going on holiday with Ben and his brother. As security queues were very long and slow that morning, we were running late so we were rushing through the airport. I was using the travelators to try and get to our departure gate as quickly as we could. Ben did not like using escalators or travelators. He always hesitated at the beginning and I was worried he would trap his toes as the conveyor belt slid under the teeth at the end. I was looking ahead, hurrying and trying to jolly Ben along as we rushed to get our flight. I was unaware that as we got off the end of a travelator, Ben expertly pressed a sequence of buttons and turned it off. This made him happy as he could get off more easily as the movement stopped, but it was maddening to the people behind us. I was not aware of what he was doing until we had gone quite a distance and along a number of travelators. An angry member of staff ran up to me and told us off! All I could do was apologise and I tried to explain that my son had done this, and hoped there weren't too many people inconvenienced by it. The staff member told me that it was not possible for a child to turn off the travelator but following another reprimand, he let us go on our way. As he saw Ben do it again he believed me! I think they have now altered these at the airport!

Disappearing children are a worry for any parent, but when your child does not communicate, the situation is more difficult. I lost Ben our local library. I was trying to find a book with Nick to help him do some homework. I had Ben sitting down reading the Thomas the Tank engine books which usually kept him busy for a long time. I don't think I took my attention off him for a moment, but he had gone and I looked all around the children's section. There was no sign of him. Then I heard an announcement.

"We have a small boy in reception who does not know his name."

I knew that had to be Ben. I rushed to the entrance and there he was, crying, flapping and kicking but being held by a security guard who was not very happy about it. The security guard handed me Ben's jumper and coat. He told me that he had held on to him by his coat, Ben had shrugged out of it. Then he had him by the jumper and he did the same thing. He was a bit angry and told me that it was not his job to hold on to little boys who were too rude to even say their name! Parents should be responsible for their children at all times and this boy should be taught some manners! I don't think I have been back to that library!

Some of the downs include times when you have to focus on the difficulties; those being the difficulties your child has and also difficulties accessing the services or support for your child.

THE 'Q' FACTOR

During a period of crisis, you are invariably involved in meetings, sending letters and campaigning. When you complete benefit forms you have to focus on the challenges and the hard times; you have to write about the worst days. It becomes too easy to think about a list of difficulties or labels and difficult to remain positive and think about the child and the good times. You have to invite professionals and strangers into your personal world and family life. It can be very challenging.

Following some weeks of pressure and stress when my son was withdrawn from school, I was exhausted and emotional. I had coped with my sons challenging behaviour, his anxiety and self doubts following bullying and failing in classes at school. As we waded through the difficulties he was experiencing, it was little wonder that his self esteem was low and that we were under pressure as a family. I tried to remain understanding and keep positive for him, reminding him of the progress and the good things, but it I cracked under the pressure. After weeks of communicating and interpreting for my son, constantly mediating between him and his sister and step Dad, one evening after my son had returned to school, my husband noticed my son was anxious and behaving erratically. He asked me "what's wrong with him, why is he so stressed?" I cracked!

I felt so frustrated that I had to explain to my husband who had been there through all the difficulties and had read all the letters to the education department, social work department, health professionals, Benefits Agencies, MP and Councillors. I felt as if I had run out of words. I couldn't even say why I was upset or what was needed to make my son feel better. It becomes so hard to stay positive when you have to explain the difficulties and admit that you need help. Every day as things become more difficult, I find coping with the children's diverse needs challenging. Sadly, it is not surprising that as families affected by disability are under such pressure, marriages fail, relationships breakdown and families are torn apart.

Generally parents attend 1 open evening per year and other visits to school are for sports day, fund raising events or concerts. These are opportunities to see the positives and concentrate on achievements. Parents of children on the autistic spectrum probably have to attend school monthly, write letters campaigning for better services or support for their child. They might have to listen to other parents speaking about their child's achievements and then listen to complaints about their own child's behaviour. They observe the sophisticated behaviour of other children interacting together and then notice their own child at the edge of a group, not sure what is happening or not interested in the other children. If they are interested, then their interaction is perhaps stilted or not welcomed, as it might be too different and unpredictable.

THE 'Q' FACTOR

Living with Autism means facing your child's difference on a regular basis. It is not something you do once and put behind you. You have to face it and deal with it every day. If *you* don't accept your child and speak positively for them, who will? However, parents can get worn out and life would be so much easier if services were more readily accessible and available. I am also conscious that I probably spend too much time speaking about the difficulties and hard times. I wonder if people are actually afraid to ask how things are going, as life is generally so challenging. I try not to dwell on the tough times but focus on the things which are improving, but it is difficult to remain positive when things are so difficult.

I have a screen saver on my computer which randomly runs through a slide show of photographs. The pictures help me recall good memories - as photographs are usually taken at a positive moment. I do have some wonderful pictures, the first day my son walked to school, the first school concert when he sang a solo, the first time I had 2 children wearing the same school uniform, the first time my son played his violin with a group of other children, my 3 children together on the trampoline, my daughter holding her kitten, volunteering, the children making Christmas cakes, Christmas mornings, birthdays, pets and visits to family.

It is good to think about the good times.

Thoughts from a sibling…

By Lauren Marwick (age 9).

At school autism is hard as you might be bullied and hurt.

It is hard living with autism as my brother gets very confused a lot of the time. Then he gets stressed and he either runs away or hits himself. This makes me feel sad and angry. I would like it if my brother did not get stressed so much.

I wish that people with autism or who are different to others wouldn't get bullied. It's not their fault and it doesn't matter to me if they are different. I wish there would be no bullying in the school.

At home everyone gets cross when my brother gets stressed, and then he gets in tears when he gets upset. I feel angry and sad.

I notice at school that people with AS sometimes want to have their own way. This makes me feel sad and angry – but more angry than sad. I wish that they wouldn't want everything to be their own way and that they would let other people choose sometimes.

Even though my brother gets stressed because he has Autism, he is also very kind. Sometimes he gets the giggles and that is really funny, you can't help laughing too.

Trudy Marwick

10 worst jobs for people with autism

Taxi driver — you can't come in my taxi, I don't like….(whatever red hat, people with glasses or beards etc) or
I only drive on the white lines.

Play supervisor — it's my turn or Leave the cars in a line, don't touch them!

Bar tender — alcohol is bad for you!

Betting shop — red rum can't run it's a drink?

Personal shopper — yes, your bum does look big in that!

Analyst — he probably doesn't like you because you are ugly!

Pharmacist — don't take drugs they are dangerous!

Hypnotist — don't look into my eyes!

THE 'Q' FACTOR

TV announcer   today we are only showing
programmes I like!

Fire alarm technician   I don't like the sound of
that alarm. Turn it off!

"ASpie" Afterthoughts…

Don't you just hate it when…

You spend 2 hours watching a movie and they leave the ending open so you are expected to draw your own conclusions?

That is not helpful to people who have difficulty with imagination! My husband tells me that cliff hangers are good movies as people can imagine their own scenarios?

Open endings are so frustrating. I went through a phase as a teenager, I used to start a book and then read the last page to ensure that I would be happy that it concluded satisfactorily. If the ending was left open, I would stop reading the book as I knew I would just be frustrated and would have wasted time proceeding with reading it just to be left to make up my mind what happened in the end!

There are mistakes in continuity in tv programmes.

When watching crime dramas I spend a great amount of time scanning the periphery of the screen, I notice car number plates. I find it very frustrating when a car number plate is used on one episode for a villan and then it is used in another programme for a different character.

THE 'Q' FACTOR

The character has a dramatic change in appearance!
I lose interest in tv programmes when there is a change of actor for a character.

The camera shakes on your favourite TV programme
I have to abandon watching a programme if the camera was shaking during filming as it makes me feel sick.

Supermarkets move everything around!
It takes me months to get used to a new lay out in a supermarket. I am a creature of habit with my shopping and I write my shopping lists based on a visual tour around the supermarket. I do not find it easy when things are changed.

You don't get the jokes
Everyone else laughs, so you laugh along, but you have no idea why something is funny.

People interrupt when you are talking about your favourite subject
I guess my obsessions are not as interesting to other people.

It is also frustrating when people interrupt when you are speaking about something; it breaks the flow of thought and makes you feel that your contribution is inadequate and not interesting.

Some people find humour and pleasure in interrupting someone else's anecdote with their own wit, but it can be quite hurtful and can make you lose confidence. When it was done to me over a period of time by the same person, I avoided their company and did not have the confidence to speak at all in groups for a long time.

People stare at you because you don't follow fashion
I am very aware that I do not follow trends, I do choose my clothes because they are fashionable, but because they are comfortable and I like them.

If I try and wear fashionable items, I find it distracts me too much as I cannot tune out the feeling of the tight item or high heels which are awkward to walk in.

Shopping centre lighting gives you a head ache and makes you feel sick
Shops are places of sensory overload

People wear over powering scent
It hurts your nose

Further reading:

Attwood, T. (1998) *Asperger's Syndrome: A guide for parents and professionals.* London: Jessica Kingsley Publishers

Grandin, T. (1995) *Thinking in pictures and other reports of my life with autism.* New York: vintage books

Jackson, L. (2002) *Freaks, Geeks and Asperger's Syndrome, A user guide to adolescence.* London: Jessica Kingsley Publishers

Aston, M. (2003) *Aspergers in Love couple relationships and family affairs* London: Jessica Kingsley Publishers

Hamilton LM. (2000) *Facing Autism Giving parents reasons for hope and guidance for help* Colorado: Water Brook

Moore C. (2005) *George and Sam* London: Penguin books

Gardner N (2007) *A friend like Henry.* London: Hodder & Stoughton

Haddon M. (2004) *The curious incident of the dog in the night time* London: Vintage

Tammet D. (2006) *Born on a blue Monday A memoir of Asperger's and an Extraordinary Mind.* London: Hodder & Stoughton

Caldwell P (2006) *Finding you finding me using intensive interaction to get in touch with people whose sever learning difficulties are combined with autistic spectrum disorder.* London: Jessica Kingsley Publishers

Notbohm E. (2004) *ten things every child with autism wishes you knew.* Texas: Future Horizons

Useful Addresses and Websites

National Autistic Society
393 City Road
London EC1V 1NG
Helpline: 0845 070 4004
www.nas.org.uk

Scottish society for Autism
http://www.autism-in-scotland.org.uk/

Autism awareness
http://www.autism-awareness.org.uk

Contact a Family
209-211 City Road
London EC1V 1JN
Tel: 020 7608 8700
Helpline 0808 808 3555
Textphone 0808 808 3556
Freephone for parents and families
(Mon-Fri, 10am-4pm & Mon, 5.30-7.30pm)
e-mail: info@cafamily.org.uk
www.cafamily.org.uk

Asperger Syndrome and Adults
http://www.aspergeradults.ca/

The Challenging behaviour foundation
http://www.challengingbehaviour.org.uk/

Parent Line Plus
TEXTPHONE 0800 783 6783
Helpline 0808 800 2222
http://www.parentlineplus.org.uk/

Autism society (USA)
http://www.autism-society.org

(Paris) online autism service directory
http://www.bbi-training.co.uk/

British Dietetic Association Provides a range of
fact sheets in relation to diet including diet and
autism spectrum disorders.
www.bda.uk.com

Careers Scotland
Provides services, information and support to
individuals at all ages and stages of planning a
career.
www.careers-scotland.org.uk

Do to learn
Excellent practical educational resources.
www.dotolearn.com

THE 'Q' FACTOR

Enquire
The Scottish advice service for Additional Support for
Learning. www.enquire.org.uk

Asperger and ASD UK Online Forum. Well supported, well organised Internet support group with email discussion and bulletin boards for sharing information. Excellent practical educational resources.
www.asd-forum.org.uk

Information on benefits and disability living allowance.
www.dwp.gov.uk/lifeevent/discare

Skill Scotland
An information and advice service for young people and adults with any kind of disability in post-16 education training and employment.
www.skill.org.uk/scotland

HM Inspectorate for Education
Improving Scottish Education.
Education for Pupils with Autism Spectrum Disorders 2006
www.hmie.gov.uk/documents/publication/epasd.pdf

SIGN Executive

The Scottish Intercollegiate Guidelines Network (SIGN) writes guidelines which give advice to Heath Practitioners and patients about the best treatments that are available.
28 Thistle Street
Edinburgh EH2 1EN
Phone: 0131 718 5090 • Fax: 0131 718 5114 Website: www.sign.ac.uk

www.ingramcontent.com/pod-product-compliance
Lightning Source LLC
Chambersburg PA
CBHW031151270326
41931CB00006B/223